Living with
PANCREATIC CANCER
A Patient and Family Guide

Living with

PANCREATIC CANCER

A Patient and Family Guide

Earl J. Campazzi, Jr., M.D., M.P.H., M.B.A.
with Guilianna Johnston

Cover Designer and Illustrator
Gregory J. Del Deo

This book contains information that is intended to help the readers be better-informed consumers of health care. It is presented as general advice on health care and its related financial aspects, including health insurance. This book, audiobook and e-book are not intended to be a substitute for the medical advice of a licensed physician, the legal advice of an attorney, or the professional advice of a financial planner. This book is based on the author's experiences, research, and viewpoints. Always consult your doctor for your individual needs about any matters relating to your health or illness.

Limit of Liability/Disclaimer of Warranty: While the publisher and author have used their best efforts in the preparation of this book, they make no representations or warranties with respect to the accuracy and completeness of the contents of this book and specifically disclaim any implied warranties or merchantability or fitness for a particular purpose. Please note that medical research and treatment are ever-evolving and that this book was written is 2023. No warranty may be created or extended by sales representatives or written sales materials. The advice and strategies herein may not be suitable for your situation. You should consult with multiple professionals where appropriate. Considering the complexity of pancreatic cancer, getting multiple opinions and consulting specialists in several areas might improve your care. Neither the publisher nor author shall be liable for any loss of profit or any other commercial damages, including but not limited to special, incidental, consequential, or other damages. Readers should be aware that internet websites offered as citations and/or sources for further information may have changed or disappeared between the time this was written and when it was read.

Educational use of this book's content is defined specifically as use in classrooms, seminars, workshops, or as part of academic research. However, this privilege is exclusively extended to non-profit educational institutions, government-run schools, and 401(c)(3) professional groups recognized for their educational contributions. To use any material from this book within these settings, prior written permission from the author is obligatory.

If you're an educator seeking to utilize content from this book, please send your request for permission to mail@campazzi.com. Your request should include your name, the institution you're affiliated with, the intended purpose of use, and the scope of the material you wish to use. This process helps us ensure that the book's content is used appropriately and responsibly in educational contexts.

It's important to note that digital copies of this book cannot be shared over networks or uploaded to educational platforms without the author's express prior approval. This is to maintain the integrity of the content and its intended use.

Please be aware that unauthorized copying, even under the guise of educational use, as well as any other unauthorized use, is a violation of copyright.

Be advised that the terms and conditions outlined for educational use are subject to periodic review and updates. This ensures that our policies stay current and effective.

Lastly, we encourage ethical use and a deep respect for copyright, reinforcing the responsibility of the educational community towards intellectual property. By adhering to these guidelines, you help us maintain a balance between protecting the author's rights and supporting meaningful educational engagement with our content.

Copyright © 2024 Earl J. Campazzi, Jr., M.D., M.P.H., M.B.A.

All rights reserved. No part of this book or e-book may be used or reproduced by any means—graphic, electronic, or mechanical, including photocopying, recording, or taping or by any information-storage retrieval system—without the written permission of the publisher, except in the case of brief quotations of up to one paragraph embodied in scientific references, critical articles and reviews.

Library of Congress Control Number:
2023918476 Earl J. Campazzi, Jr., M.D., West Palm Beach, FL

ISBN: 979-8-9892184-0-0 paperback
ISBN: 979-8-9892184-1-7 hardcover
ISBN: 979-8-9892184-3-1 e-book
ISBN: 979-8-9892184-2-4 audiobook

Earl J. Campazzi, Jr., M.D.
Campazzi Concierge Medicine
440 Royal Palm Way, Suite 100
Palm Beach, FL 33480-4179
(561) 440-8879
drc@campazzi.com
www.campazzi.com

In memory of
Kevin M. Saviola

Acknowledgments

I want to thank my wonderful supporters, Dr. David and Moira Dooley. They were so encouraging, as I wrote in memory of Moira's first husband, Kevin M. Saviola. He was a superb man. Like so many, he lost years and his retirement to this brutal disease.

I would also like to give a special thank you to Steven and Brooke Schonfeld for their generous gift to the Pancreatic Cancer Network (PanCAN).

Donna Manross, Vice President, and Ana Gonzalez, Manager II, of PanCAN, graciously arranged for the patient quotations from pancreatic cancer survivors, KH, AS, and JG. I especially want to thank these survivors for giving to other patients by adding their voices of experience to my book.

I appreciate the kind words of my great friend and excellent physician colleague, Dr. Nabil Tadross. He practiced medicine for many years with Cleveland Clinic in Cleveland, Ohio, before being recruited to Cleveland Clinic Florida.

Earl J. Campazzi, Jr., M.D., M.P.H., M.B.A.

Gregory J. Del Deo is an exceptional commercial artist skilled in illustrations, book cover design, and graphic creation. Despite my frequent changes, he remained professional and patient. I highly recommend his services. You can reach him via email at deldeo@gmail.com.

Four-leaf clover emojis to Jimmy Dunne who taught me that if I didn't engage my readers with stories, my message would be lost.

The beautiful layout of my book was crafted by the talented team at BookNook.biz. A special thanks goes to Zvonimir Bulaja, Judith Bardera, and the owner, Kimberly "Hitch" Hitchens, for their exceptional work.

I would like to thank three attorneys and a line/copy editor who reviewed sections of this book. They wish to remain anonymous.

For the first version of this book, five wonderful friends and colleagues spent a lot of time helping make it better for you, the readers:

- Dr. Dana R. Krumholz is a retired hospice and palliative care physician. She excelled at helping people who were very sick or who were nearing the end of their lives. She also stepped in as an early editor, saving the last edition which helped guide this one.

- Dr. Allyson Ocean is an Associate Professor at Weill Cornell Medical College and is an expert in pancreatic cancer. She also started the pancreatic cancer charity, Let's Win PC.

- Jon S. Saxe is a very experienced pharmaceutical and biotechnology executive who has served as a director of over twenty-five companies.

- Dr. Nicholas S. Aradi is a psychotherapist who works with cancer patients and their families in South Florida. He is an expert in cognitive behavioral therapy as well as in trauma processing and resolution. He spent many hours helping me with the emotional and psychological aspects of treatment.

- Dr. Gregory E. Merti is my medical school classmate and a medical director for Sentara Health Plans, a health insurer. He added essential information about health insurance, which is so important to understand.

Many thanks to Dr. Bert Vogelstein at Johns Hopkins for kindly discussing genetic testing and medication choices with me on a Saturday. As a Professor of Oncology at the Ludwig Center and a leading figure in cancer research, his insights were invaluable. I'm deeply grateful for his time.

This book would not have been possible without the assistance of my summer intern, Guilianna Johnston. She is an intelligent and hardworking young woman with wisdom and judgment beyond her years. She will be an excellent physician.

Last but most, the love and support of my wife, Julie, guided me through this project. Julie is not only beautiful but also a caring, intelligent and creative woman.

Foreword

Getting a diagnosis of pancreatic cancer is undeniably a pivotal experience. You may be left with an abundance of questions whilst trying to understand your diagnosis and having to traverse an unfamiliar array of treatment options. However, Dr. Earl Campazzi provides a comprehensive resource for patients in Living with Pancreatic Cancer to begin their journey with pancreatic cancer empowered with knowledge.

Dr. Campazzi is not just a physician, but an advocate and a source of unwavering support for those touched by this disease. He is a prime example of a physician who approaches patient care both wholly and completely, extending a compassionate hand to his patients not just medically, but also through education and empathy. Living with Pancreatic Cancer emphasizes the need for a collaborative approach to patient care, as patients need to be the drivers in their health journeys and should be equipped with the knowledge to do so.

In this book, the information transcends the medical textbooks and research databases and there is a focus solely on you and your journey navigating this disease head-on. Within these pages, you will discover how to make informed decisions on your healthcare, and how to utilize the tools available to you, and you will be reminded that you are never alone. In a world where pancreatic cancer is often overshadowed by fear, your journey deserves to be circumscribed by hope and resilience.

Nabil Tadross, M.D.
Head of the Concierge Medicine Practice in Fort Lauderdale, Cleveland Clinic Florida
Board Certified in Internal Medicine
Clinical Assistant Professor of Medicine at the Cleveland Clinic Lerner College of Medicine, Case Western University of Medicine

Introduction

Pancreatic cancer is extremely unfair. Nobody should have to suffer from it. Pancreatic cancer can be overwhelming for patients and their loved ones. It is vital to have reliable access to information and resources to help navigate the diagnosis and treatment. I hope this book provides helpful insights and support for you.

There could be many reasons why you are reading or listening to this book. Perhaps you have recently been diagnosed with pancreatic cancer or are seeking help during the later stages of the disease. Maybe you're reading this because you care about someone or are helping to care for them. Additionally, those with pancreatic cancer are often worried about the possible increased risk of the disease for their children and grandchildren.

If you find out you have pancreatic cancer, you're probably very worried and not sure what to do next. While it is important to trust and follow your doctor's recommendations, it is also essential to make informed decisions. As a primary care provider, I offer a broader perspective than your oncologist. I also can provide guidance on difficult topics such as when to seek a second opinion, getting additional tests, and optimizing your care. The goal is to ensure you receive the best treatment currently available to keep you healthy until breakthroughs are discovered.

To help you read only the parts that matter to you, I made a special table of contents titled "How Your Book Applies to You." It has a short, italicized summary of each chapter. This will help you decide if a chapter is helpful for your situation.

Please note, this work is an expanded and extensively revised edition of my 2017 book, *Just Diagnosed™ with Metastatic Pancreatic Cancer: First Steps and More.*[1]

Artificial intelligence (AI) can be a valuable tool in treating pancreatic cancer, a key idea I want to highlight in this book. In four different ways, I use AI: firstly, for searching references; secondly, for generating text that I subsequently quote; thirdly, for transforming my writing when it is complex and technical into simple, easy-to-read sentences; and fourthly, for acting as an editor to put the finishing touches on the book.

Sadly, there is no secret or miracle cure for metastatic pancreatic cancer at the time I am writing this book. While it's natural to focus on what we don't know yet, what really matters is how your current treatment compares to the best options available today. The top care, including specific diagnosis and initial treatment plans, can often be found at a specialized cancer hos-

---

1. Campazzi, E. J. (2017). *Just Diagnosed™ with Metastatic Pancreatic Cancer: First Steps and More.* Suzanne Wright Foundation.

pital, an academic medical center. A pancreatic cancer survivor makes this point for us:

> I went to Memorial Sloan Kettering Cancer Center in New York when I was first diagnosed. My older son was working there at the time, and he got me an appointment in a timely manner. I believe that I'm alive today because of that visit. **JG**

The book's most important reference, which I recommend you search online and read, is "Why a Top Cancer Center Could Save Your Life."[2] It is difficult to explain why the quality of medical care varies widely across communities in the United States.[3]

The case of Supreme Court Justice Ruth Bader Ginsburg shows us the benefit of excellent medical care. "She had no symptoms of the disease at the time—it was discovered during a regular checkup."[4] This was amazing since "there is no screening

---

2. Begley, S. (2009, October 16). Why a top cancer center could save your life. *Newsweek.* http://www.newsweek.com/why-top-cancer-center-could-save-your-life-81425, accessed May 14, 2023.

3. Miranda, E. (2014, February 1). Unwarranted variations in care: Searching for sources and solutions. *Journal of Ethics | American Medical Association.* https://journalofethics.ama-assn.org/article/unwarranted-variations-care-searching-sources-and-solutions/2014-02

4. Reynolds, K. (2020, September 25). U.S. Supreme Court Justice Ruth Bader Ginsburg dies of complications from pancreatic cancer. *Pancreatic Cancer Action Network.* https://pancan.org/news/u-s-supreme-court-justice-ruth-bader-ginsburg-dies-of-complications-from-pancreatic-cancer/

test for healthy adults for pancreatic cancer,"[5] per MD Anderson, one of the best cancer centers.

How did her doctor diagnose her at such an early stage? Her doctors were undoubtedly excellent and spent time with her. Perhaps they ordered a scan to check on her previous colon cancer.[6] Everyone should have this level of care.

Justice Ginsburg had surgery that went perfectly, but about eight years later, her cancer came back. She was treated again at Memorial Sloan Kettering and Johns Hopkins. Many say she lived with pancreatic cancer for over ten years because of her great doctors and strong will to fight.

Getting outstanding healthcare can make a big difference. It might not be possible to get the same quality of care and, especially, the same access as the members of the Supreme Court, but you can still aim for the best. This means searching for the top doctors and places that often handle pancreatic cancer.

It might be difficult to get a timely appointment with the doctor of your choice. The quote above tells us that the patient got an appointment quickly because their son worked at Memorial Sloan Kettering Hospital. Another patient shared, "My hus-

---

5. Underferth, D. (2019, November 6). Can you screen for pancreatic cancer? *MD Anderson Cancer Center*. https://www.mdanderson.org/publications/focused-on-health/can-you-screen-for-pancreatic-cancer-.h20-1592991.html

6. City of Hope. (2020, July 20). 5 things we can learn about cancer from Justice Ruth Bader Ginsburg. *CancerCenter.com*. https://www.cancercenter.com/community/blog/2020/07/ginsburg-cancer-learn

band found a very respected surgeon and tried to get an appointment with him. Unfortunately, we were unable to schedule the doctor we wanted." **KH** Luckily, she was able to get an appointment with a surgeon at MD Anderson because her son was a district manager at a major pharmaceutical firm. Later in the book, there are methods to get urgent doctor appointments.

Given the seriousness of pancreatic cancer, it is essential to avoid mistakes. One example is the case of Steve Jobs, one of the world's most intelligent and creative people. He was co-founder of Apple. In October 2003[7], he was diagnosed with a rare type of pancreatic cancer known as neuroendocrine[8,9] or islet cell tumor, which accounts for only 7%[10] of cases. This is the best type of pancreatic cancer since it can often be cured through surgery. Patients with this type of cancer also tend to survive for longer than those with the most common type, adenocarcinoma.[11]

---

7. Greenlee, H., & Ernst, E. (2012). What can we learn from Steve Jobs about complementary and alternative therapies? *Preventive medicine*, 54(1), 3-4. https://doi.org/10.1016/j.ypmed.2011.12.014

8. Harmon, K. (2011, October 7). The puzzle of pancreatic cancer: How Steve Jobs did not beat the odds—but Nobel winner Ralph Steinman did. *Scientific American*. https://www.scientificamerican.com/article/pancreatic-cancer-type-jobs/

9. Greenlee, H., & Ernst, E. (2012). What can we learn from Steve Jobs about complementary and alternative therapies? *Preventive Medicine*, 54(1), 3-4. https://doi.org/10.1016/j.ypmed.2011.12.014

10. American Cancer Society. (2022, January 14). Key statistics for pancreatic neuroendocrine tumor. https://www.cancer.org/cancer/pancreatic-neuroendocrine-tumor/about/key-statistics.html

11. Yadav S, Sharma P, Zakalik D. Comparison of Demographics, Tumor Characteristics, and Survival Between Pancreatic Adenocarcinomas and Pancreatic Neuroendocrine Tumors: A Population-based Study. *Am J Clin Oncol*. 2018 May; 41(5): 485-491. doi: 10.1097/COC.0000000000000305. PMID: 27322698.

In Steve Jobs' case, surgery was necessary for effective treatment. However, he chose to ignore his doctor's advice. He attempted to treat his cancer with acupuncture, dietary supplements, and juices.[12] Despite the strong suggestions of his family and friends, he refused surgery because he did not want to have his body subjected to the procedure. This may have been due to a belief in "magical thinking"—that if he ignored the cancer, it would disappear.[13] Eventually, Jobs underwent surgery nine months after his initial diagnosis in 2004.[14]

It was too late to cure him because his cancer had already spread. At that point, Jobs completely changed his approach and began searching for any available medicine or experimental science to help him. He was among the first individuals to have his entire genetic code sequenced. He even traveled to Switzerland to try experimental treatments. Tragically, it was too late to save him, as his slow-growing pancreatic cancer had already metastasized. He passed away on October 5th, 2011.[15]

---

12. Walton, A. G. (2011, October 24). Steve Jobs' cancer treatment regrets. *Forbes*. https://www.forbes.com/sites/alicegwalton/2011/10/24/steve-jobs-cancer-treatment-regrets/

13. Walton, A. G. (2011, October 24). Steve Jobs' cancer treatment regrets. *Forbes*. https://www.forbes.com/sites/alicegwalton/2011/10/24/steve-jobs-cancer-treatment-regrets/

14. Greenlee, H., & Ernst, E. (2012). What can we learn from Steve Jobs about complementary and alternative therapies? *Preventive Medicine, 54*(1), 3-4. https://doi.org/10.1016/j.ypmed.2011.12.014

15. The Economic Times. (2022, October 4). A decade after Steve Jobs' death, has Apple lost its magic? https://economictimes.indiatimes.com/magazines/panache/a-decade-after-steve-jobss-death-has-apple-lost-its-magic/articleshow/86753764.cms

How Your Book Applies to You

When I write about pancreatic cancer, I often use the pronoun "you." This is because I'm talking directly to the people with pancreatic cancer. If you're reading this for someone else, I hope you understand why I chose my words to speak directly to those who have pancreatic cancer.

I've put in quick overviews for every chapter so you can easily find what matters most to you. I know your time is important.

Acknowledgments ix
Thank you to many and to more than I can name.

Foreword xiii
Dr. Nabil Tadross, Cleveland Clinic Florida

Introduction xv
Your strategy should be to get the best possible care currently available, enabling you to wait for better treatment.

Hope 1

Advances in treatments, testing your tumor in the lab, stimulating your immune system, and analyzing the results with AI all give hope that breakthroughs seen in other cancers are coming.

Advice from Fellow Pancreatic Cancer Patients 19

No one can advise you like a fellow patient.

Basics About Your Pancreas and Pancreatic Cancer 25

Information is power. You need to understand your problem.

Step Zero: Biopsy 41

A doctor who is a specialist, called a pathologist, can find out details about your pancreatic cancer which can improve your care. They do this by examining a tiny piece of your tumor under a microscope and testing it in other ways. Also, they can collect live cancer cells to grow into an organoid.

Step Zero+: Send Your Cells to Grow an Organoid 45

Organoids are little pieces of your tumor that are kept alive. Scientists grow these in a lab. They use organoids to see how different medicines, or combinations of drugs, work against your tumor. This way, doctors can figure out which treatments might help you the most.

Step One: Pause 47

After you find out you're sick, it's really important to spend some time—but not too much—to learn more about your illness. It's a good idea to get advice from more than one doctor to help decide what kind of treatment you want. Usually, waiting about two weeks before starting your treatment is seen as safe and enough time.

Step Two: Choose Your Team 49

People who have had pancreatic cancer before say that having a team helps a lot and in many ways.

Step Three: Get Organized 71

You will need help getting and staying organized. The volume of medical and financial records can be overwhelming. Knowing a single fact or finding a trend can be important to your health.

Step Four: Choose Your Oncologist 77

There are several things to keep in mind—your gut feelings, does he or she discuss anything besides chemotherapy, their education, any language barrier, and if their medical license/certifications are valid.

Steps Five, Six and Seven: Pathology, Radiology and Oncology Second Opinions (Start asking for appointments at the same time—get in any order) 81

Usually, a cancer doctor who specializes in pancreatic cancer adds the most. However, a mistake or new finding in radiology or pathology can be a game changer.

Step Eight: Surgery, If Possible 93

By far, the best chance to cure pancreatic cancer is surgery. The words "if possible" are very important. Sometimes, an experienced surgeon will operate when other surgeons say no.

Step Nine: Consider a Biopsy for an Organoid Before Starting Treatment................................111

Having an organoid gives you a big advantage. Potentially, it could be lifesaving.

Step Ten: If Surgery Was Not an Option or Your Cancer Came Back After Surgery, Choose Your Treatment....................................... 119

Chemotherapy is the most common choice but there are alternatives.

Step Eleven: Monitor for Depression & Anxiety and Consider Mental Health Care 153

It might sound strange, but it's possible to have pancreatic cancer without always feeling sad.

Step Twelve: Engage Palliative Care 165

Research shows that patients do better if their symptoms and treatment side effects are addressed from the beginning.

Step Thirteen: Avoid Falling (AI assisted)[16] 167

Falls can be a double whammy if you have pancreatic cancer. You are more likely to fall, and it's harder to get better after a fall. It's really important to try not to fall because falls can be painful, make you bedridden, and even be deadly.

---

16. OpenAI. (2023). ChatGPT [Computer software]. Retrieved from https://www.openai.com/

Step Fourteen: Use Home Nursing and Other Supportive Services 173

My thirty-plus years of medical practice have taught me that being at home with a nurse and family provides the most comfort when someone is seriously ill.

Step Fifteen: Living with Pancreatic Cancer

Managing Day to Day 183
Work 185
Travel 188
Doing Your Own Research 190
Participating in Clinical Trials 200
Healthy Living 204
Family Risk 218

Financial Aspects

Understanding and Dealing with Health Insurance 233
Federal Governmental Support 246
State Government Resources 253
Tapping into Little-Known Funds 255
What Non-Profits Offer 267
Dip Into Your Rainy Day Fund 274
Estate Planning 274

Summary 277

Appendix A: Websites to Verify Medical Licenses .. 279

Appendix B: Definitions and Abbreviations 287

Afterword **293**

About the Intern **295**

About the Author **297**

Doctors need to understand what's happening in the real world. They should know the different problems and unfair situations their patients might face. We help people with pancreatic cancer who may have extra challenges. These include people whose primary language is not English, who can't hear well, who can't see, or who have little money. More support makes it easier for patients to get the help they need, like taking tests and talking to experts.

Certainly, racial disparities exist in American healthcare and are a matter of concern. Although finding solutions to these disparities falls outside my area of expertise, I am fully aware of the significance of this issue and the urgent need to address it.

When we talk about pancreatic cancer, it's really important to know that "the incidence of pancreatic cancer is higher in African Americans than in any other racial group in the United States... African Americans are more often diagnosed with advanced, and therefore, inoperable cancer."[17] This might be partly because they smoke more, which can lead to pancreatic can-

---

17. Pancreatic cancer and African Americans. Pancreatic Cancer and African Americans—Pancreatic Cancer—Johns Hopkins Pathology. (2023). https://pathology.jhu.edu/pancreas/familial/about/african-americans

Living with Pancreatic Cancer: A Patient and Family Guide

cer.[18] But a big problem is also getting medical care late. This is probably because of issues with access and the availability of medical care in African American communities, which can be deadly and shorten lives.

No matter how much money someone has, I do my best to help them get the cancer treatment they need. Getting the best medical care can cost a lot, but I can guide you on how to find help even if you have little money.

If you are poor, you have to try extra hard to get good medical care. This might mean asking charity groups for support or joining special research projects called clinical trials. These options can take a lot of time to figure out. This book gives you helpful information on how non-profits can help people with pancreatic cancer. It also offers tips on finding money to help pay your medical bills.

In this book, we use the symbols $, $$, $$$, and $$$$ to show how much different groups of people can pay for healthcare on their own. I'll help you figure out what medical tests and services are good for you. For example, spending a few hundred dollars to double-check your pathology test results is really important for everyone. But having a nurse always with you at home is something only rich people can afford.

$—It's challenging or even impossible for people in this group to pay for the parts of their bill their health insurance doesn't

---

18. Pancreatic cancer and African Americans. Pancreatic Cancer and African Americans—Pancreatic Cancer—Johns Hopkins Pathology. (2023). https://pathology.jhu.edu/pancreas/familial/about/african-americans

cover, called the deductible and copayment. Being sick often means the person can work less, or not at all, so they're earning less money. This makes it even harder to deal with money issues. If they're lucky, they might have a few hundred dollars saved up to pay for any care or tests that your insurance won't cover.

$$—Apart from paying for the necessary costs of treating pancreatic cancer, people in this group also have an extra amount, somewhere between $1,000 and $10,000. This extra money could be used wisely for additional treatments, tests, and scans, and seeking advice from other doctors.

$$$—If this is your group, you can pay some money from your pocket for pancreatic cancer treatments. However, there are limits to how much you can spend. You could have between $10,000 to $100,000 available for this.

$$$$—If additional treatment or nursing can help and you are lucky enough to be in this group, you have the money to pay for it. You can also donate money to help find a cure for pancreatic cancer or give to a charity that helps people with the disease.

Hope

Magic Johnson, born Earvin Johnson, Jr. on August 14, 1959, is often considered one of the best basketball players ever. During his 13-year career with the Lakers, he made it to the All-Star Game ten times, won the NBA championship five times, and was named the Most Valuable Player (MVP) three times.

In a shocking press conference in November 1991, Johnson announced that he was HIV-positive and would retire from professional basketball. When he made his announcement, treatment choices were not as effective, and there were fewer options than today.

In the early 1990s, the main way of treating HIV and AIDS was to control symptoms and stop or treat any extra infections. HIV weakens the immune system, which can lead to infections. This meant people needed antibiotics, antifungals, antiviral drugs, and other treatments.

The first medicine to fight against HIV, called zidovudine or AZT, was approved by the US Food and Drug Administration (FDA) in 1987. This medicine works by stopping the virus from making copies of itself in the body. But even though AZT was a significant advance in treating HIV, it wasn't a cure and had severe side effects.

After discovering he was sick, Magic Johnson started taking AZT. About five years later, there was a medical breakthrough. Magic was able to switch to more effective combination therapies. Eventually, there was a dramatic drop in the number of people dying from AIDS. Now, people with HIV can live long and healthy lives with the help of HAART drugs.

In August 2015, President Jimmy Carter, the 39th president of the United States, discovered he had a severe illness called metastatic melanoma. Doctors found cancer in his liver and soon confirmed it was malignant melanoma. After more tests, they discovered the cancer had spread to his brain in four spots.

He was already 90 years old. Because the disease was severe and he was advanced in age, the outlook or prognosis was bad. Metastatic melanoma usually has a low rate of people surviving. When it spreads to the brain, that outlook is typically even worse.

Despite the odds, Carter began aggressive treatment, including surgery, radiation therapy, and a groundbreaking immunotherapy drug called pembrolizumab (Keytruda). Pembrolizumab is a checkpoint inhibitor, which essentially works by enabling the immune system to recognize and attack cancer cells more effectively.

Remarkably, the former president's treatment was successful. As of December 2015, just a few months after his diagnosis, Carter announced he was cancer-free. His doctors found no evidence of the four brain lesions, and his liver showed no signs of the disease, reflecting a significant improvement in his condition.

Since then, President Carter has remained active, attending church, teaching Sunday school, and participating in charitable causes through the Carter Center. His resilience and the success of his treatment have offered hope and inspiration to many battling cancers worldwide.

It is important to note that Keytruda, the drug used to treat President Carter, can also treat certain individuals with pancreatic cancer. A blood test can determine whether it can benefit you.

Sadly, Keytruda is proven to work for only a small group of pancreatic cancer patients, around 1% to 3%.[19] But for these, it can extend their lives from about a year and a half to even a few more years.[20]

There are different ways to bring hope to those with pancreatic cancer today. One key idea is that we don't always need a

---

19. Ahmad-Nielsen, S. A., Bruun Nielsen, M. F., Mortensen, M. B., & Detlefsen, S. (2020). Frequency of mismatch repair deficiency in pancreatic ductal adenocarcinoma. *Pathology, Research and Practice, 216*(6), Article 152985. https://doi.org/10.1016/j.prp.2020.152985
20. Kahl, K. L. (2021, January 31). Long-term follow-up shows Keytruda continues to improve survival in patients with PD-L1-positive advanced NSCLC. *Cure Today.* https://www.curetoday.com/view/long-term-follow-up-shows-keytruda-continues-to-improve-survival-in-patients-with-pd-l1-positive-advanced-nsclc

total cure. It's a good outcome if we can control and handle the symptoms of pancreatic cancer. Think about AIDS. We don't have a cure yet, but the treatments available are so good that people living with AIDS can usually continue their usual lives. The same thing applies to conditions like high blood pressure, type 2 diabetes, and many heart problems.

Of course, we would rather have a cure. What gives me hope is a special way of finding the best cancer medicine for each person. This is known as personalized medicine. My idea is to use artificial intelligence to find what is the best treatment for each person with pancreatic cancer.

Everyone's pancreatic cancer is a little different. These zoomed-in pictures below show pancreatic cancer cells and tell us key things. These cells do not look alike. This makes it important for a pathologist to sort them accurately. The left cell, even though it's cancerous, looks more like a normal cell and seems to be growing slower. The right cell, on the other hand, is growing very quickly. It's making a lot of a certain protein that acts like a fake ID, tricking our body's defense system. It might be possible to create a special treatment tailored just for this type of cancer cell.

So, think of pancreatic cancer as both one disease and a group of different diseases. As we said before, using a complete plan or system is the best way to make real progress. It's better than depending on just one medicine.

Even small changes can make a big difference:

Living with Pancreatic Cancer: A Patient and Family Guide

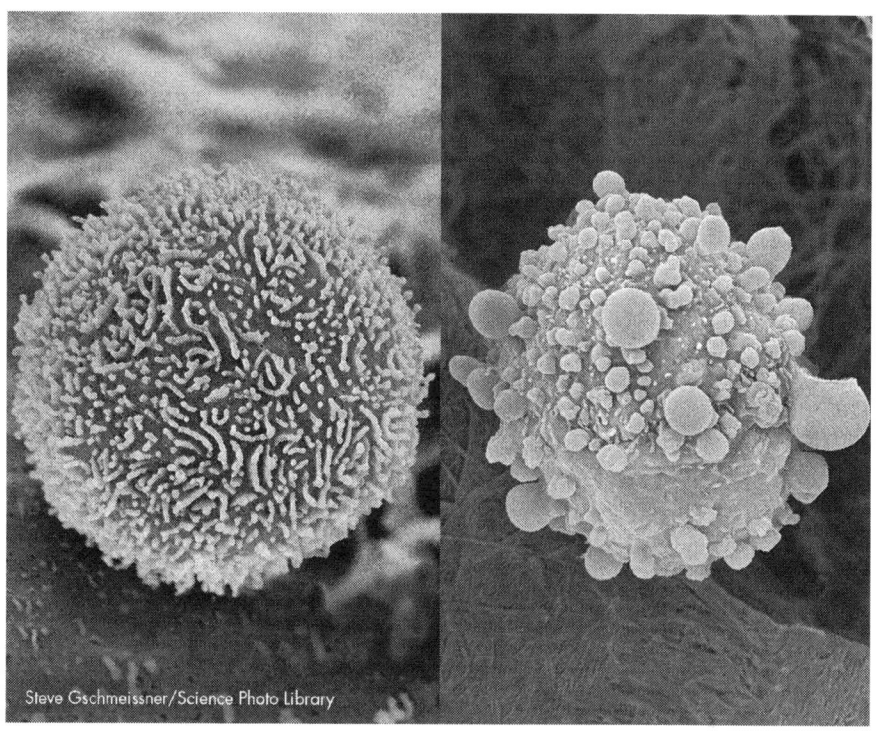
Steve Gschmeissner/Science Photo Library

Although the chemo that was recommended was the same chemo my health care provider in California recommended, MSK [Memorial Sloan Kettering Cancer Center, New York, NY] had done a recent clinical trial in which they found the chemo was as effective at 85% as it was at 100%. The issue was that particular chemo at 100% was so toxic that most people couldn't tolerate it. I believe that I'm alive today because of that visit. **JG**

AI can help us figure out what similar small changes to make, but let's first learn about it and what it can do. The April 16, 2023 edition of Sixty Minutes tells about AI and chess:

5

Scott Pelley:
Bard [the name of a Google AI program] appeared to possess the sum of human knowledge... with microchips more than 100,000 times faster than the human brain... AlphaZero [the name of another Google AI program] ... dreamed up a winning chess strategy no human had ever seen...
But this is just a machine. How does it achieve creativity?

Demis Hassabis:
It plays against itself tens of millions of times. It can explore parts of chess that human chess players and programmers who program chess computers haven't considered.

Scott Pelley:
It never gets tired. It never gets hungry. It just plays chess all the time.

Demis Hassabis:
Yes, it's amazing, because you set off AlphaZero in the morning, and it starts playing randomly. By lunchtime, it's able to beat me and beat most chess players, and then by the evening, it's stronger than the world champion.[21]

AI is also doing some exciting work in biology, especially with proteins. First, let's understand what proteins are. They're like long strings made from smaller parts called amino acids.

---

21. Cetta, D. S., & Brennan, K. (2023). The AI revolution: Google's developers on the future of artificial intelligence—60 Minutes [Video]. YouTube. https://youtu.be/880TBXMuzmk

Imagine a necklace made from different kinds of beads. In a protein, you usually have 50 to 200 of these "beads," or amino acids.

These amino acids have special qualities that make the protein fold into a 3D shape. Think of it as like turning a straight string of beads into a twisted, folded sculpture. The shape of this "sculpture" is really important for how the protein works in our bodies.

Figuring out these shapes has been very difficult. Just knowing the order of the amino acids has not been enough to guess what shape the protein will take. But in 2020, an AI program named DeepMind did something amazing. It could predict the shape of proteins from only the order of the amino acids as accurately as expensive and time-consuming experiments to determine their shapes.[22] By 2022, it had figured out the shapes of all 350,000 the proteins that we know are in the human body.[23]

AI isn't magical; it requires data to learn and then operate effectively. AI is like a detective—it's good at spotting clues or patterns. It can help find connections in large sets of data.

We need more information about pancreatic cancer for AI to really help us. The best way to get this is by studying organ-

---

22. Service, R. F. (2020). 'The game has changed.' AI triumphs at protein folding. Science, 370(6521), 1144-1145. DOI: 10.1126/science.370.6521.1144
23. Callaway, E. (2022). 'The entire protein universe': AI predicts shape of nearly every known protein. *Nature, 608*(7921), 15-16. https://doi.org/10.1038/d41586-022-02083-2

oids.[24] An organoid is a mini-version of your tumor made of your cells kept alive in a science lab. High-throughput screening with many drugs and drug combinations are used on these organoids to see which one best kills your cancer cells.

Scientists can make organoids from cancer cells collected from patients during a biopsy. A biopsy is when doctors take some cells from your pancreas to check for cancer. Then, a pathologist uses a microscope to examine these cells closely. This helps to determine if the person has cancer or not, and which type. Even though it's pretty simple to get live cells during the biopsy, keeping them alive and bringing them to a research lab requires a lot of careful planning.

At UF Scripps Florida, they are using high-speed machines to do high-throughput testing on organoids. In their lab, they can test pancreatic cancer cells with 1,536 different kinds of drugs and mixes of drugs very quickly.[25] This creates so much information that AI is needed to analyze it. Soon, AI will learn from organoid data to read tumor DNA, quickly picking the best treatment.

By checking out how medicines, including chemotherapy, work on the organoids, scientists can choose a treatment or mix

---

24. Robinson, K. (2022, May 26). Patient-derived organoids predict chemotherapy efficacy for pancreatic cancer. *Cell Science from Technology Networks*. https://www.technologynetworks.com/cell-science/articles/patient-derived-organoids-predict-chemotherapy-efficacy-for-pancreatic-cancer-362019

25. Spicer, T. (2023). High-throughput molecular screening center. *The Herbert Wertheim UF Scripps Institute for Biomedical Innovation & Technology*, Scripps Biomedical Research, University of Florida. https://scripps.ufl.edu/departments/centers-and-specialties/high-throughput-molecular-screening-center/

of medications that work best on your tumor in the lab. This method could help treat cancer in a way specific to each person. But even though it's moving forward quickly, it's still being tested and isn't regularly used by doctors yet. Refer to Step Nine to discover a list of scientists working with organoids, understand the process of creating an organoid from your own cancer cells, and gain additional information.

The other way we can treat pancreatic cancer is by strengthening your immune system. Your immune system was not strong enough to fight your cancer (maybe it stopped other cancers you never knew about) as it grew. You cannot rely only on it to treat your pancreatic cancer. However, improving your immune system can still be helpful in your treatment. Too often in medicine we dismiss something helpful if it is not the total solution.

First, let's explore the potential of the immune system and then look into how artificial intelligence could potentially boost its effectiveness. The precise role of the immune system in fighting cancer and its variability among individuals remains a topic of discussion among health care professionals and scientists. Attempts have been made to strengthen the immune system by extracting blood, treating it in a lab, and then returning it to the body.[26] This approach, though, is expensive and time-consuming.

British cancer researchers say, "the immune system can help fight cancer. Some immune cells can identify and destroy

---

26. DeSelm, C. J., Tano, Z. E., Varghese, A. M., & Adusumilli, P. S. (2017). CAR T-cell therapy for pancreatic cancer. *Journal of Surgical Oncology*, 116(1), 63-74. https://doi.org/10.1002/jso.24627. Epub 2017 Mar 27. PMID: 28346697; PMCID: PMC5491361.

cancer cells."[27] Learning more about and improving the immune system of pancreatic cancer patients has great potential:

- Weak immune systems in mice and humans often lead to higher cancer risk.

- Organ transplant patients who are taking drugs to lower their immune responses are more likely to develop cancer.

- People with HIV-1, which weakens the immune system, are more at risk of cancer.

- The amount and strength of immune cells found in human tumors can predict a patient's chances of survival.

- Cancer cells have mutations that the immune system can recognize.

- Specific immune cells can recognize and eliminate cancerous cells.

- A possible cancer treatment could be strengthening the patient's natural immune response by blocking specific immune proteins.[28]

---

27. Cancer Research UK. (2020, July 7). The immune system and cancer. https://www.cancerresearchuk.org/about-cancer/what-is-cancer/body-systems-and-cancer/the-immune-system-and-cancer
28. Corthay, A. (2014). Does the immune system naturally protect against cancer? *Frontiers in Immunology, 5*, Article 197. https://doi.org/10.3389/fimmu.2014.00197. PMID: 24860567; PMCID: PMC4026755.

Again, AI needs information to find out how to strengthen each person's immune system. It's not as easy as it sounds. Our body's immune system is truly complicated. We already have many tests to see how it's doing.[29] The tests mentioned below have a role in immune system functioning and are all available today:

- Your DNA is not exactly the same as your tumor's DNA. Both have about 20,000 to 25,000 genes,[30, 31] but slight yet important differences exist. New Amsterdam Genomics is already using AI to analyze genetics testing results.[32] According to AI, understanding which genes are actively expressed (being used) by searching for gene-specific RNA is more important to know than merely identifying the genes that exist. This process is referred to as epigenetics.[33]

- Immune system function

- Tumor markers

---

29. Institute of Medicine (US) Committee on Military Nutrition Research. (1999). C, Overview of immune assessment tests. In *Military Strategies for Sustainment of Nutrition and Immune Function in the Field*. National Academies Press (US). https://www.ncbi.nlm.nih.gov/books/NBK230966/
30. U.S. National Library of Medicine. (2023, March 22). What is a gene? *MedlinePlus Genetics*. MedlinePlus. https://medlineplus.gov/genetics/understanding/basics/gene/
31. Genome.gov. (2022, August 16). A brief guide to genomics. https://www.genome.gov/about-genomics/fact-sheets/A-Brief-Guide-to-Genomics
32. New Amsterdam Genomics. (2023). New Amsterdam Genomics is powerful insightful life-changing. https://www.nagenomics.com/
33. OpenAI. (2023). ChatGPT [Computer software]. Retrieved from https://www.openai.com/

- Gut Microbiome[34]. "With 70-80% of immune cells being present in the gut... it is increasingly recognized that the gut microbiome also affects systemic immunity."[35] In simpler terms, the tiny organisms living in your gut can both help and harm your body's ability to fight off diseases. It's important for us to learn more about this.

- Hormones

- Vitamins

- Micro-nutrients (tiny elements or substances needed for normal growth and development)

- How fast drugs are processed in your body (Cytochrome P450 monooxygenases)

- Peptides[36]

- Telemedicine, wearable health trackers and digital health tools are becoming more common. These tools are espe-

---

34. Zheng, D., Liwinski, T., & Elinav, E. (2020). Interaction between microbiota and immunity in health and disease. *Cell Research, 30*, 492-506. https://doi.org/10.1038/s41422-020-0332-7
35. Wiertsema, S. P., van Bergenhenegouwen, J., Garssen, J., & Knippels, L. M. (2021). The interplay between the gut microbiome and the immune system in the context of infectious diseases throughout life and the role of nutrition in optimizing treatment strategies. *Nutrients, 13*(3), Article 886. https://doi.org/10.3390/nu13030886
36. Wang, L., Wang, N., Zhang, W., Cheng, X., Yan, Z., Shao, G., Wang, X., Wang, R., & Fu, C. (2022). Therapeutic peptides: Current applications and Future Directions. *Signal Transduction and Targeted Therapy, 7*(1). https://doi.org/10.1038/s41392-022-00904-4

cially useful for tracking how patients feel and respond to treatments in real-time. AI suggested this bullet point.[37]

To help your body fight pancreatic cancer, a variety of drug and supplement combinations can be used. First, we need to check how well your immune system is currently working, your genes and other factors listed above. We don't have tests for everything, so we'll focus on the ones we can test for. Using AI, we can determine the optimal blend of supplements, medications, and vaccines to support your immune system as it helps you fight pancreatic cancer. While people take supplements to boost their immune system, to my knowledge, no one is doing extensive testing and using AI to pick the best combination for each patient from the long list above.

Finally, we can keep an eye out for any signs that the cancer is coming back by using a special blood test called a liquid biopsy[38]($$) and treat it quickly if it does. AI isn't just for choosing treatments. It can also estimate the chances of cancer returning in patients and suggest the best schedule for follow-up tests.[39]

The test, named Galleri®, is made by a company called Grail. It's the only one like it that has full approval from the FDA and

---

37. OpenAI. (2023). ChatGPT [Computer software]. Retrieved from https://www.openai.com/
38. Heredia-Soto, V., Rodríguez-Salas, N., & Feliu, J. (2021). Liquid biopsy in pancreatic cancer: Are we ready to apply it in clinical practice? *Cancers (Basel), 13*(8), Article 1986. https://doi.org/10.3390/cancers13081986. PMID: 33924143; PMCID: PMC8074327.
39. OpenAI. (2023). ChatGPT [Computer software]. Retrieved from https://www.openai.com/

is widely available. Other companies are trying to create similar tests because this technology still has room for improvement.[40]

Liquid biopsy is a simple blood test that can find small traces of pancreatic cancer cells and their DNA. This helps doctors know early on if your cancer is coming back, making it easier to treat. This test is also good for early detection of pancreatic cancer in those who are at high risk for getting cancer, such as family members of a cancer patient. For the foreseeable future, Doctors will also keep using special medical pictures like mammograms, CT scans, and MRIs to check if the cancer returns.

To summarize my plan which simply brings together the work of so many in the cancer field:

1. Greatly decrease the size of tumors with surgery, chemotherapy or radiation therapy or a combination of.

2. Treat the remaining cancer:

    A. Personalized chemotherapy guided by AI

    B. Personalized immune strengthening guided by AI

3. Monitoring for recurrence with tumor markers, liquid biopsies and imaging.

4. Treat any recurrences as appropriate.

---

40. Galleri® Test. (2023a). Test performance: Deeper dive for health care providers. https://www.galleri.com/hcp/galleri-test-performance

We can improve the way we fight pancreatic cancer by using organoids, applying high-throughput methods, and using AI to analyze all data. This is a bold statement, but it is supported by scientific literature. In, "The potential of AI to improve cancer care is only going to grow," the European Society for Medical Oncology writes:

> In the field of cancer genetics, for example, many of the mutations included in modern genomic reports used to match patients with targeted therapies were identified by AI tools comparing the genetic profiles of hundreds of thousands of patients and making predictions about their role in the development of cancer.[41]

In, "Machine learning and AI in cancer prognosis, prediction, and treatment selection: A critical approach," Dr. Zhang and his colleagues write, "Artificial intelligence (AI), which is used to predict and automate many cancers, has emerged as a promising option for improving healthcare accuracy and patient outcomes. AI, itself, summarizes, "So, these examples show that AI is really changing the way we handle cancer, making it clear that it helps a lot in finding, treating, and improving the health of cancer patients."[42]

---

41. European Society for Medical Oncology. (2023, November 20). The potential of AI to improve cancer care is only going to grow. *Cancer Health*. https://www.cancerhealth.com/article/potential-ai-improve-cancer-care-going-grow

42. Zhang, B., Shi, H., & Wang, H. (2023). Machine learning and AI in cancer prognosis, prediction, and treatment selection: A critical approach. *Journal of Multidisciplinary Healthcare, 16*, 1779-1791. https://doi.org/10.2147/JMDH.S410301

Doctors' guiding principle is, "do no harm." However, given pancreatic cancer's 5-year survival rate of approximately 13%,[43] caution must give some ground to urgency. This balancing act between caution and urgency is not just a medical challenge but a moral imperative, as every percentage point increase in survival rates represents lives extended, families preserved, and hope fostered.

The speed of medical research, specially making new drugs, is purposely slow. Initial promising results often do not work out. Sometimes, there are side effects so severe that using the medicine is not smart or ethical. However, what I purpose involves using data from existing medicines and proven laboratory tests. The use of AI in medicine, especially pancreatic cancer should proceed as Cox said, "with a quantum leap."[44]

If patients with pancreatic cancer don't join forces to raise funds and demand immediate action, the use of AI in advancing research and treatment will move forward slowly. "... any field dealing with human health, caution is warranted alongside enthusiasm and therefore, newer technologies like AI, machine learning, and big data analytics are introduced more slowly and

---

43. Pancreatic Cancer Action Network. (2024). Five-year survival rate for pancreatic cancer increased to 13% signaling more progress and more hope for patients. https://www.pancan.org
44. Cox, B., & Coustasse-Hencke, A. (2023, October 16). AI is revolutionizing oncology with a quantum leap in cancer treatment. *Pharmacy Times*. https://www.pharmacytimes.com/view/ai-is-revolutionizing-oncology-with-a-quantum-leap-in-cancer-treatment

more cautiously than in other sectors."[45] Zhang and his colleagues point out the issues:

- Data Privacy

- Fragmented Data

- Knowledge Graphs

- Scale

- Data Normalization

- Complicated Data[46]

These are all legitimate concerns to which I add fear of lawsuits, unclear funding/profit motive and just inertia.

Addressing the technical and legal problems with AI does not have to be a slow process like approving a new drug. None of the issues above require experiments or mice, observing patients over time to see if it is effective and what its side effects are.

---

45. European Society for Medical Oncology. (2023, November 20). The potential of AI to improve cancer care is only going to grow. *Cancer Health*. https://www.cancerhealth.com/article/potential-ai-improve-cancer-care-going-grow

46. Zhang, B., Shi, H., & Wang, H. (2023). Machine learning and AI in cancer prognosis, prediction, and treatment selection: A critical approach. *Journal of Multidisciplinary Healthcare, 16*, 1779-1791. https://doi.org/10.2147/JMDH.S410301

Like it does for drugs the Food and Drug Administration (FDA) has to approve for critical applications directly affecting patient care. For example, FDA oversight is typically required to ensure patient safety and efficacy of the AI tool for cancer diagnosis or treatment decisions, However, FDA approval for AI is usually faster than it is for new drugs.

Not every use of AI in healthcare needs to get the green light from the FDA. For instance, when doctors use AI to get a clearer picture of medical data like lab tests, there's no need for FDA approval of the AI program. In simpler terms, if doctors rely on AI to help make decisions by interpreting information, the AI doesn't require FDA approval. However, when AI takes on a more active role, such as adjusting how fast medication is delivered through an IV pump, then it must be approved by the FDA.

Using AI data analysis to improve the treatment of pancreatic cancer is a big task that can't be done by just one doctor. It requires a team of experts and the use of patient data. But this kind of project wouldn't cost as much as finding a new cancer medicine. Funding could come from the government, a charity, or a company, and a university hospital could carry out the research. A private company might be the best choice to fund it because they usually respond the quickest to new opportunities.

I really hope everyone sees just how powerful AI can be. We need to start using it quickly and in many different ways to make treating pancreatic cancer better and more successful.

Advice from Fellow Pancreatic Cancer Patients

1. **Based on your experience, what resources/information would you suggest people just diagnosed with pancreatic cancer access?**

   After I was diagnosed, I just went into this awful, negative attitude that my life was over. My mother passed away 20 years earlier from pancreatic cancer. When I was diagnosed, it was a time of high-profile cases—Patrick Swayze, Randy Pausch. I had only heard of a death in relation to this disease and it took my daughter to find this website [Pancan.org] and print off 50+ testimonies of people with survivor status. That gave me hope and "Hope" is what is needed to turn your mind from death to life and give a person the courage to fight. I did not personally use the option to talk with the caller network, but as somebody who has been taking calls since I got through my treatment and surgery (around 14 years' worth of calls), I certainly understand this amazing resource provided to people where they get answers to their fears. **KH**

Survivor stories and experience. Get the right treatment and make the treatment work by following what the survivors do. This includes a healthy diet and a positive attitude. I will recommend not giving up and trying to survive first. **AS**

In addition to the Pancreatic Cancer Network, I would recommend going to the Seena Magowitz Foundation Warrier Page. There are numerous stories from survivors offering hope to those struggling with this disease. **JG**

2. **If you or your loved one went to a national cancer center or sought a second opinion from a pancreatic cancer expert physician, please reflect on that process and how much it helped you.**

I did both a second and third opinion.

It was hard to go so far away from home. We were fortunate that we had some close acquaintances in Houston so it wasn't totally a foreign feeling, but I would be away from my family, friends—people all necessary to give me moral support. We were looking at a huge financial commitment. It wasn't so much the cost of the treatment and surgery (we were fortunate that my husband had retired from the Army, and we had great insurance in Tricare and had a supplemental plan to pick up anything Tricare did not cover), but it was also the cost of renting a furnished apartment while I completed my treatment protocol.

Dr. Evans let me do some of the treatment in Spokane and worked well with my oncologist there. However, when we came to the radiation, he would not waver on demanding I complete that in Houston. He felt his team was the best qualified to do the radiation. We weren't arguing. Faith is strong for both me and my husband and I felt that guided us in all our decision making. We lived in Houston for two months while I finished the treatment and then went home to recuperate for a month. I went back at the end of the month and completed the surgery. **KH**

3. **How did you or your loved one keep going with normal life despite pancreatic cancer—please include practical advice about more rest/modified schedules as well as dealing with the emotional aspects?**

The following quotes highlight that everyone's journey is different. Even though you can learn a lot from other people, remember that you are special, and your own path will be one-of-a-kind:

At the beginning, I was exhausted from the disease, and I had a lot of building my body back up. The month prior to my actual diagnosis, I had been losing a pound a day. In a month, I lost about 35 lbs. I was fortunate that I worked for a school district as a social worker. I received my diagnosis about two weeks after we broke for summer vacation.

It was a time of reflection for me while I watched my friends go back to work. My world was different—not worse —just different. I was fortunate that I had little reaction to the chemo. I sat in a chair while they administered the chemo "cocktail" for five hours. My family usually brought lunch to me. I never got sick from it, and I didn't lose my hair (both things I had been very scared about—I even cut my hair short so I wouldn't be as shocked when I started losing it. It did get thinner, but I was probably the only one who noticed.) **KH**

My mom raised me all by herself since I was ten. She took a lot of responsibilities in life. When she was diagnosed, I told her not to worry about anything. I will take care of all, including getting groceries, cooking, etc. My mom was able to rest well and just relax every day, without worrying about anything. It was in 2020, there was not much we could do for entertainment. She just watched drama. Most of the time, she felt like a normal person and forgot about the condition. I suggest that she not research anything online and keep a positive attitude. That was also the year I started believing in the law of attraction. Positive thinking is critical. **AS**

The first six months were very difficult, and I didn't enjoy a normal life. I had difficulty eating and keeping any food down. After that time, I found that rest was the key to handling the difficult chemo. Small meals were also important as large meals would overwhelm me. **JG**

4. **How did you balance important family events and the desire to travel with your treatment schedule? Looking back, would you make the same choices?**

When things got tough, I simply let my family know and with grace and love they met my needs. I felt pretty good, but had to make some adjustments to sleeping arrangements, etc. Everybody understood and I just powered through. I felt extremely loved and coddled. I was strong when I was able and let them help when I felt it was a good balance and also felt that they needed to understand I wasn't always going to be at my best. There was no guilty conscience or pushing myself to be more than I felt like being. **KH**

I would have chemo on Monday and go home with a pump pack that would be removed on Wednesday. Thursday was always my worst day and many times I didn't get out of bed. By Saturday I would feel well enough to travel. Periodically, I would take a chemo holiday when I was going to be gone longer than a week. I wouldn't change a thing. **JG**

5. **What type of support from friends and family was the most helpful—conversation, notes, phone calls, or did you prefer to keep things private?**

Before leaving for M.D. Anderson in Houston, we had a huge party in our backyard. We called it the "Kick Cancer's Ass" party. We invited my work colleagues, my husband's, friends near and far, the neighborhood. We had more than

100 people show up to give well wishes by signing a banner to take with me.

I had friends and family bring me lunch while I sat for five hours in the chair getting my chemo cocktail. I have never felt so loved and cared for and most of all blessed. It was the best of times, and it was the worst of times, but I wouldn't change any of it. I never felt the need to keep any of it private. If people wanted to help, we found small ways to let them—my family is very self-sufficient. My only regret was that we didn't really have the Catholic parish attachment at the time. We had been so busy with careers; we had neglected our faith. But that led me to making a commitment to myself that if I got through this challenge, I would give back in any way I could to help others. I've kept that commitment for the last 13 years by taking calls for pancan.org and M.D. Anderson. **KH**

We shared with only a few friends. Due to Covid, we decided to just accept emotional support from a few people instead of any physical support. We didn't share this with anyone else, nor any of our family members as their worries or questions probably wouldn't help the situation. **AS**

I was fortunate enough to have great support from family and friends. What was most helpful was when I met a five-year survivor of Stage IV Pancreatic Cancer. It was this individual whom I met one year after my diagnosis who made me realize that survival was even an option. I told her that if I survive this, I wanted to do for others what she did for me. **JG**

Basics About Your Pancreas and Pancreatic Cancer

Your pancreas is a six-inch organ that looks like a hot chili pepper lying at an angle. Here, it is shown with and without a tumor.

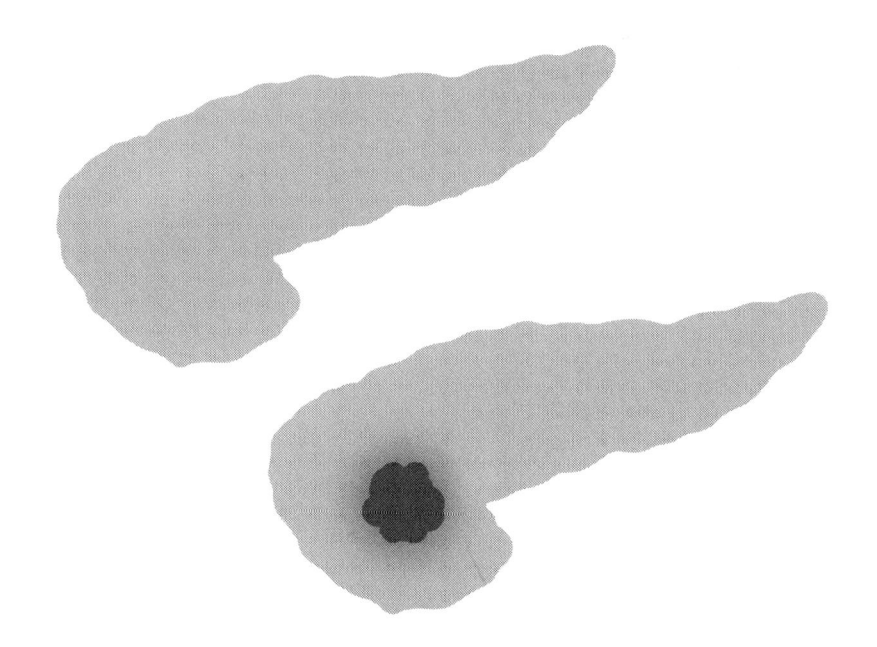

Your pancreas is an organ in your body that has two main jobs: it helps break down the food you eat, and it helps control the sugar levels in your blood. It is located at a diagonal angle behind your stomach and below your breastbone.

The central part of the pancreas is slightly to the right side, while its tail goes up toward the left side behind your stomach. It is shielded by the lower left ribs to keep it safe.

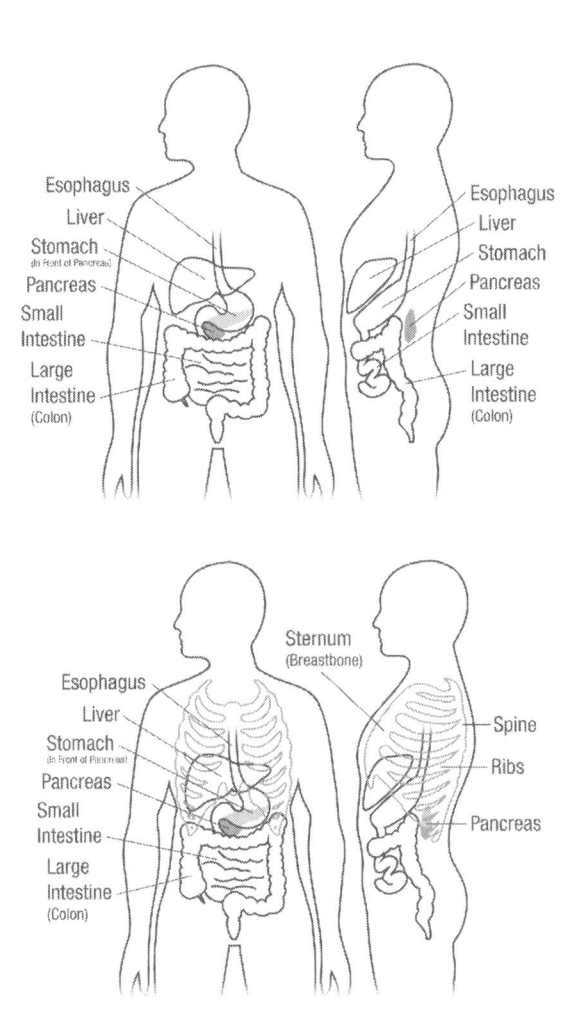

The pancreas is tricky because it is in the middle of the body. This can cause problems when trying to find and treat pancreatic cancer. Since the pancreas is deep inside, doctors can't feel it when they examine a patient. Once the tumor has gotten much bigger, they will notice that the area over your pancreas feels sensitive or sore. This makes it challenging to diagnose and treat problems with the pancreas.

Sadly, sometimes neither the patient nor their doctor notices that a lump in the pancreas as it grows until it becomes too large to remove by surgery or effectively treat. Treating pancreatic cancer using surgery and radiation therapy is challenging because the tumor is close to important blood vessels with high pressure called arteries. If these blood vessels are accidentally cut during surgery, they can bleed heavily.

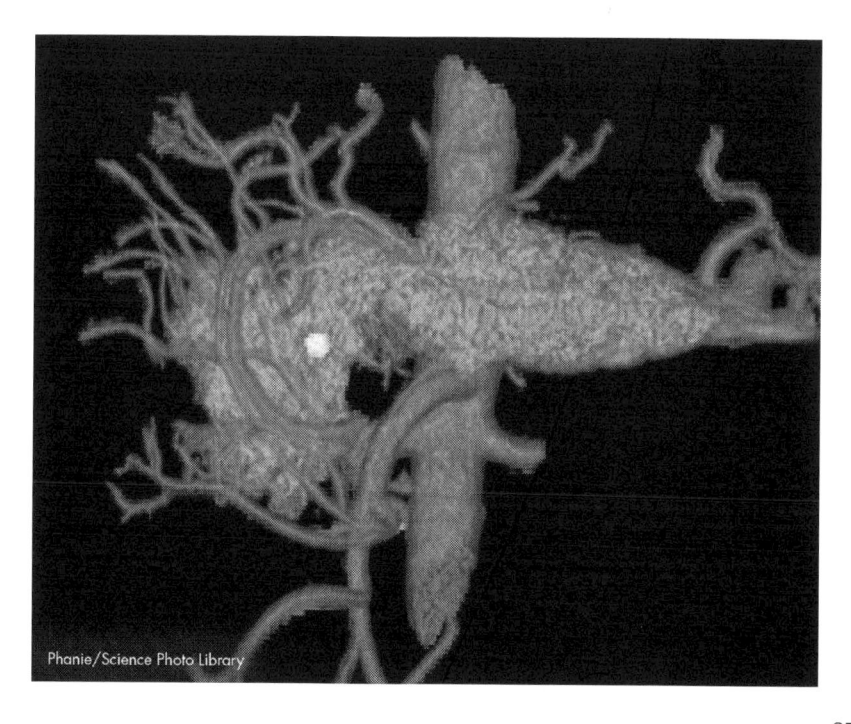

Phanie/Science Photo Library

Take a moment to think about your whole body. Understanding how it works will help you make smart choices about treatment. The human body is so complex that it is amazing that it works and works so well. It makes sense that treating such a complex system is not easy. Be careful when you hear about simple cancer cures because there is nothing simple about the body. Also, almost every treatment works better for some than for others and has unintended negative effects called side effects.

Think about your body like it's a map on Google. This map can zoom in or out at four different levels. The amount of detail you can see changes a lot at each level. You can look at the entire earth, a map of your state, your neighborhood, and a picture of your house. Now, let's use this idea for your body, looking at it in four different levels of zoom:

1. **Whole person:** It is so easy to start by focusing on the cancer. However, the medical care team and the family must remember that they are treating a person with pancreatic cancer, not simply pancreatic cancer. Any cancer treatment must also concern itself with the health and well-being of the person. This is a reminder to look through the broadest lens first.

2. **Organs:** Your body is made up of different parts that are called organs. We can only see these organs with special tools like X-rays, ultrasounds, CT scans, or MRI scans. Doctors can also see them during surgeries. These organs are like different sections in a big store, each doing only a few tasks.

A. Some organs are extra important. We call them vital organs because we need them to stay alive. An example is your liver. Your liver is like a big cleaning machine for your body. It removes harmful chemicals that we eat, drink, or that our body produces. For instance, your liver is what "sobers you up" after drinking alcohol.

The liver is a pretty tough organ. Even when pancreatic cancer spreads to the liver, causing many giant tumors, the liver can still do its job. But there's a point where the cancer can make the liver stop working. Sadly, getting a new liver won't help to cure pancreatic cancer. The new liver would quickly get cancer, too, and stop working. Many times, people with pancreatic cancer pass away because their liver fails.

B. Your pancreas is another organ in your body. It's been giving you some problems, but it's not a vital organ like your liver. This means you can live even if your pancreas is removed. If pancreatic cancer spreads to the liver, it's usually considered incurable. In such cases, even if surgery on the pancreas is possible, it would be for symptom relief, not a cure.

3. **Cells:** A lot is happening inside each cell, much like a bustling city. Mostly, cells use their DNA, like a set of instructions, to create three different types of proteins.

A. Enzymes: Imagine these like automatic robots. When a cell in your pancreas releases an enzyme, it has one specific task that it does repeatedly. Some enzymes, for instance, chop up the protein we consume into little parts so we can absorb it. Others help to transform the fat in our food so our bodies can absorb and use it.

B. Hormones: Hormones are unique proteins produced by specific cells in the pancreas and released into the bloodstream. They act as messengers for other cells. For instance, insulin, a hormone produced by the pancreas, will be discussed further, including its functions.

C. Cell-surface markers refer to proteins outside cells, such as those in the pancreas. There are two primary types of these markers.

    a. Cell surface identity markers are like ID badges for cells. They are proteins that tell the body's defense cells, "Hey, I'm a part of the body, don't attack me!" For example, they let these defense cells know that pancreas cells are friends, not foes.

    Understanding the differences between these tags is really important. Some cancer medicines work better because they are designed to target specific markers or proteins on the surface of cancer cells. As time passes, we're getting better at creating treatments specifically targeting your cancer cells. Again, this is personalized medicine, and it can make a big difference in how well your treatment works.

> b. Hormone receptors are also present in pancreatic cancer cells. These receptors are proteins geared explicitly toward a hormone, like a lock and key. These receptors can also be targets for cancer drugs.

4. **DNA:** DNA is a special code or instructions that tell our cells what to do. This code is stored inside each of our cells and makes us who we are. For example, every cell in our pancreas contains information from three billion pairs of letters from this DNA code. They are like the zeros and ones of data in computer software. Each cell has as many DNA pairs as water drops in three swimming pools! But here's the hard part: cancer happens when mistakes occur in this DNA code and the cancer cells multiply to become many, many cells. Because of this, trying to stop cancer from spreading is a considerable challenge.

The pancreas lets out the proteins it makes in two ways. One way is by sending hormones straight into your bloodstream. The other way is by sending enzymes to your intestines through a tube inside your pancreas called the pancreatic duct.

Surprisingly, most pancreatic cancers begin in the simple cells that form the pancreatic duct. The most common kind of pancreatic cancer, called adenocarcinoma, happens when something goes wrong in these cells.

When cells in the ducts of the pancreas change into adenocarcinoma, it can cause a big problem. Cancer can block the path of digestive enzymes. As mentioned above, these enzymes are like little automatic cutting machines that break down food into tiny pieces to help digestion. It can be very dangerous if these enzymes can't get out, and start building up inside the pancreas. Too many enzymes can begin to hurt the pancreas and the tissues around it.

If there's a blockage inside our body, doctors can place a stent to help. A stent is a small, folded metal tube that pops open like a spring once it's in place. Then the small tube that helped place the stent is pulled back and out of the body. It's used to open a tube in our body known as the bile duct. This helps with the functioning of the pancreatic duct. The pancreatic duct is typically too small for a stent. But by placing a stent in the larger and downstream bile duct, we can stop too many enzymes from building up.

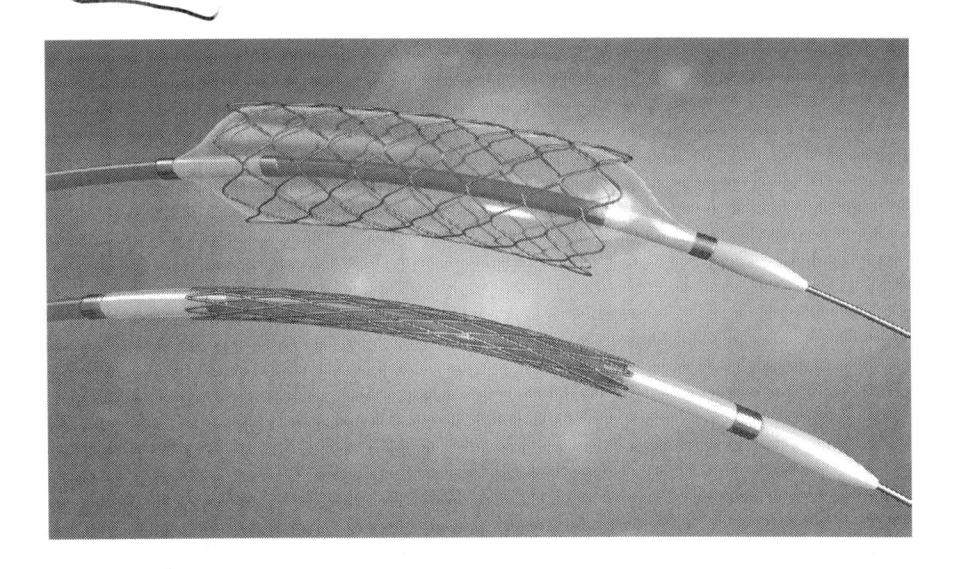

iStock. (n.d.). [Image number 114169089] [Photograph]. Accessed September 10, 2023, from https://www.istockphoto.com/

When pancreatic cancer of the adenocarcinoma type gets worse, it can hurt the cells in the pancreas that make hormones. The body's most important hormone is insulin, which helps our cells take in sugar from the blood for energy. The medical term for this type of sugar is glucose.

A decrease in insulin for any reason is a disease called diabetes. If you don't have enough insulin, sugar can't get where it needs to go—inside your cells. Think of insulin as carrying glucose from your bloodstream to the inside of your cells. You might feel hungry or weak because your cells need sugar to work properly. It is a little confusing as blood sugar levels go up while cells do not have enough. "This is like having a lot of food on the table, but not being able to eat it."[47] AI explains.

Sometimes, cutting down on sweets in your diet can prevent diabetes or help control it if you're already dealing with this health issue. It's like putting less fuel on a fire to keep it from getting too big. Diabetes is a condition where your body has difficulty processing sugar, so eating less, especially carbohydrates, can make a big difference.

Pancreatic cancer is a very serious illness, but not all pancreatic cancers are the same. There are some rare kinds called neuroendocrine and acinar cell carcinoma. These are names for special cells in the pancreas where these kinds of cancer begin.

---

47. OpenAI. (2023). ChatGPT [Computer software]. Retrieved from https://www.openai.com/

Steve Jobs, whom I mentioned in the Introduction, had neuroendocrine pancreatic cancer. Acinar cell carcinoma and neuroendocrine carcinoma (also known as pancreatic endocrine cancer or islet cell carcinoma) are usually found before spreading to other parts of the body. They're pretty uncommon, each making up only 1-2% of all pancreatic cancer cases.[48, 49] People with these rare pancreatic cancers do better compared to those with pancreatic adenocarcinoma. Surgery is usually used for both.

From AI, here is more about them:

Where They Come From:

- **Neuroendocrine Carcinoma:** Comes from special cells in the pancreas that make hormones like insulin.

- **Acinar Cell Carcinoma:** Comes from cells that make juices to help digest food.

- **Pancreatic Ductal Adenocarcinoma:** Comes from cells that line the tubes in your pancreas.

---

48. Calimano-Ramirez, L. F., Daoud, T., Gopireddy, D. R., Morani, A. C., Waters, R., Gumus, K., Klekers, A. R., Bhosale, P. R., & Virarkar, M. K. (2022). Pancreatic acinar cell carcinoma: A comprehensive review. *World Journal of Gastroenterology, 28*(40), 5827-5844. https://doi.org/10.3748/wjg.v28.i40.5827. PMID: 36353206; PMCID: PMC9639656.

49. American Cancer Society. (2023, January 13). Key statistics for pancreatic neuroendocrine tumor. https://www.cancer.org/cancer/types/pancreatic-neuroendocrine-tumor/about/key-statistics.html

How Common They Are:

- **Neuroendocrine Carcinoma:** Pretty rare.

- **Acinar Cell Carcinoma:** Even rarer.

- **Pancreatic Ductal Adenocarcinoma:** The most common type, making up about 85-90% of all pancreatic cancers.

Signs and Symptoms:

- **Neuroendocrine Carcinoma:** Stomach pain or hormone problems like low blood sugar.

- **Acinar Cell Carcinoma:** Usually stomach pain, weight loss, and yellow skin (jaundice).

- **Pancreatic Ductal Adenocarcinoma:** Like Acinar—stomach pain, weight loss, and jaundice.

What They Look Like Under a Microscope:

- **Neuroendocrine Carcinoma:** Shows up as hormone-making cells.

- **Acinar Cell Carcinoma:** Shows up as digestive juice-making cells.

- **Pancreatic Ductal Adenocarcinoma:** Shows up as cells from the tubes in the pancreas.

How to Treat Them:

- **Neuroendocrine Carcinoma:** Usually removed with surgery. Special medicines can also help.

- **Acinar Cell Carcinoma:** Surgery is the first choice. Specific drugs are used for severe cases.

- **Pancreatic Ductal Adenocarcinoma:** Surgery, chemotherapy, and sometimes radiation are used. It's harder to treat than the other types.

Chances of Getting Better:

- **Neuroendocrine Carcinoma:** Generally, people do better with this type than with other kinds of pancreatic cancer.

- **Acinar Cell Carcinoma:** People usually do a bit worse with this type than with Neuroendocrine but better than with Ductal Adenocarcinoma.

- **Pancreatic Ductal Adenocarcinoma:** Unfortunately, this type usually has the worst outlook of the three.

Where They Spread:

- **Neuroendocrine Carcinoma:** Often spreads to the liver.

- **Acinar Cell Carcinoma:** Can spread to the liver, lungs, and nearby glands.

- **Pancreatic Ductal Adenocarcinoma:** Usually spreads to the liver, lungs, and other organs and is generally more aggressive.

Do They Make Hormones?

- **Neuroendocrine Carcinoma:** Sometimes makes hormones that cause specific symptoms.

- **Acinar Cell Carcinoma:** Usually doesn't make hormones.

- **Pancreatic Ductal Adenocarcinoma:** Also usually doesn't make hormones.

So, each type comes from different cells in the pancreas, has different symptoms, and needs different treatments. The most common type is Pancreatic Ductal Adenocarcinoma, but all of them need quick attention from doctors.[50]

---

50. OpenAI. (2023). ChatGPT [Computer software]. Retrieved from https://www.openai.com/

Pancreatic cancer cells are like criminal gang members that can move to different bodily places through our blood. They can go to places like the liver (where they usually go), lungs, bones, brain, and other parts. We hope the cancer doesn't spread to many places in the body. But sadly, it does.

When pancreatic cancer moves to a different part or parts of the body, it is known as "metastasized." This means the cancer has probably also spread in very small, hard-to-see ways throughout the body. To find these tiny cancer spots, doctors use a special machine called a PET (Positron Emission Tomography) scanner. The only way to treat these tiny cancer spots is with chemotherapy, which travels all through your body. This is called systemic treatment.

Cancer is a sickness that makes cells grow and split apart without stopping. Usually, the number of cells in our body grows in two steps. First, the cells get bigger, and then they split into two separate cells. This happens most frequently before we are born as we go from 1 cell to billions of cells. There is slower growth in childhood. But cancer cells are different. They turn on the growth genes, which are the instructions that our bodies used when we were young. This leads to cancer cells growing and dividing very quickly, but they are also abnormal and don't work the way they should.

Another reason your immune system struggles to fight pancreatic cancer because cancer cells make web-like shields, like spiderwebs, called fibrous stroma (see back cover photo). This shield helps the cancer cells grow by protecting them from your immune system.

The net-like structure around your pancreatic cancer cells can greatly slow blood flow. Yet, unlike other kinds of cancer, pancreatic tumors can live with even a small amount of blood. The fact that the tumor has a minimal blood flow helps the cancer cells fight off treatments. This happens because blood carries chemotherapy and other drugs; if there's less blood flow, only a tiny amount of the drug can reach the cancer cells.

Step Zero: Biopsy

I named this Step Zero because not everyone should or will have a biopsy. A biopsy is a medical process where doctors take a small piece of an unusual growth in your body and examine it under a microscope. They do this to find out if you have pancreatic cancer. It's a starting point in understanding what's going on in your body. Some of the readers of this book may have already experienced this procedure.

Whether or not you need a biopsy for a suspicious mass that could be pancreatic cancer depends on several things. These include the characteristics of the mass, the symptoms you have, and the results of other tests. The biopsy gives a definite diagnosis by studying your tumor sample under a microscope. This information is crucial for deciding on the best treatment plan.

With the help of AI, here are some reasons why a biopsy might be done:

1. To confirm the presence of cancer and find out the type and stage of the cancer.

2. To get information about the genetic makeup of your cancer cells, which helps choose the proper treatment.

3. To see how well the cancer treatment has worked; the doctors can adjust it if needed.

However, there are situations where a biopsy may not be necessary, such as:

1. When imaging tests like CT, MRI, or PET scans clearly show that it is cancer, no further confirmation is needed.

2. A surgeon plans to remove your tumor and believes it can be done entirely. In that case, they might skip the biopsy and examine the tissue after surgery to confirm cancer presence.

3. Doctors may find other ways to diagnose cancer if a patient's health cannot handle a biopsy.

Remember that every person's situation is different, so decisions about whether to do a biopsy should always be made together with a health care provider who knows your health history and current condition well.[51]

---

51. OpenAI. (2023). ChatGPT [Computer software]. Retrieved from https://www.openai.com/

Another concern about biopsy is spreading the disease while trying to treat it. Needle track seeding is when the needle inserted into your tumor spreads your cancer as it is being pulled out. In my opinion, the importance of getting a biopsy when your doctor recommends it far exceeds this risk which is estimated to be in the range of 0.003% (1 in 33,000) to 0.4% (1 in 250).[52] "When focusing on pancreatic adenocarcinoma... [a biopsy is] without an apparent [negative] impact on prognosis."[53]

---

52. Archibugi, L., Ponz de Leon Pisani, R., Petrone, M. C., Balzano, G., Falconi, M., Doglioni, C., Capurso, G., & Arcidiacono, P. G. (2022). Needle-Tract Seeding of Pancreatic Cancer after EUS-FNA: A Systematic Review of Case Reports and Discussion of Management. *Cancers, 14*(24), 6130. https://doi.org/10.3390/cancers14246130
53. Archibugi, L., Ponz de Leon Pisani, R., Petrone, M. C., Balzano, G., Falconi, M., Doglioni, C., Capurso, G., & Arcidiacono, P. G. (2022). Needle-Tract Seeding of Pancreatic Cancer after EUS-FNA: A Systematic Review of Case Reports and Discussion of Management. *Cancers, 14*(24), 6130. https://doi.org/10.3390/cancers14246130

Step Zero+: Send Cells from Your Biopsy to Grow an Organoid

People often connect the phrase "Plus it" to Walt Disney. This phrase means he liked to go beyond the normal—taking it to max.[54]

Organoids are the "plus," the best idea in your book. We talked about them in the Hope chapter. When I talk to my patients, sometimes they ask, "Doctor, what would you do if your family member had pancreatic cancer?" One of my answers would be to have them ask for an organoid.

This is a great way to see which treatments might work before they are used in a patient. It helps us find the best treatment faster. This way, we can fight the disease more effectively and give our loved ones the best chance to improve.

---

54. McKinney, P. (2020, November 27). Walt Disney's "Plus It" approach to better ideas. *Killer Innovations*. Retrieved July 12, 2023, from https://killerinnovations.com/walt-disneys-plus-it-approach-to-better-ideas/

Step Nine shows how to arrange an organoid with the centers doing organoid research.

Step One: Pause

There are various ways you could have learned that you have pancreatic cancer. The best case is having had no pain or symptoms before an incidental finding. For example, doctors can discover a tumor in the pancreas during a scan checking for a different problem, most commonly gallbladder disease. When pancreatic cancer is found this way, it is often relatively good news because there is a higher chance that it has not yet spread to other parts of the body.

Most commonly, you do not know you have pancreatic cancer until you have symptoms. It can be like getting ready to ride a roller coaster. At first, you feel a little queasy, like a bellyache. It doesn't seem like much, but it sticks around. You start to worry, like how you feel as you climb up the first big hill of the coaster.

You decide to see your regular primary doctor. The doctor orders some standard tests. The test results are a bit worrisome, like when you're going higher and higher on the roller coaster. Fear of not knowing is intense when a CT scan is needed, more so than the thought of the first drop on a roller coaster. When they find a lump in your pancreas on the CT scan, it feels like the scary rush of dropping down the first hill on the roller coaster. Everything feels like it's happening too fast and out of your control.

When you're on a roller coaster, you can't suddenly stop it. But when dealing with pancreatic cancer, you have some control. You can think of it like having an emergency brake. This is a scary disease, and getting diagnosed with it can feel like a shock. You'll need time to understand what's happening, gather facts, undergo additional testing, get second opinions, and decide on your first treatment. But remember, you shouldn't take too much time because it is important to start treatment quickly.

One of the first questions is the length of time you can safely spend gathering information and seeking second opinions before beginning treatment. It would be best if you asked the physician who made your diagnosis how urgently you need treatment. If your physician initially responds with "as soon as possible," you should ask whether this is an emergency that requires treatment today or this week or whether two weeks would be a safe and reasonable time to gather information before making a treatment decision.

The books and articles tell us that pancreatic cancer usually takes about ten years to grow from just one cell. When we finally notice it through medical tests or symptoms, it is growing a lot faster than it did at the beginning. Normally, waiting about two weeks or more to start treatment is okay. But, again, for emphasis, it's always a good idea to talk to your cancer doctor about when to start treatment since they know your situation best.

Step Two: Choose Your Team

If you have pancreatic cancer, you're going to have to tackle a tough and exhausting plan for treatment. You'll have to make many choices, even when feeling sick.

When you find out you have pancreatic cancer, you might feel like you should take care of yourself. You may want to be in control and not ask for help from others. However, people who have gone through pancreatic cancer before advise using a team-based approach. They recommend this because dealing with cancer is a big job, and there may be times when you don't feel your best, physically or mentally. Having a team is about getting help, not about losing control. Let's take a look at how the KH's family did things right after they found out about the cancer:

> With the diagnosis, my family immediately went into Team H mode. Each member seemed to find their niche. My daughter became my cheerleader. She put signs up everywhere in the house saying "30+" which was the length of time I needed to expect to still live. My son became my

researcher, taking time to find the most recent news surrounding pancreatic cancer. My husband became everything else—my daily supporter, my comforter, my plus-1 when I went to all my doctor appointments. **KH**

It's really important to put together a group of people to help you during this time. This group should include doctors, family members, friends, and even hired helpers. This team will focus on three main goals:

1. To make sure you receive the top-level health care you need. This includes:

    A. Most effective treatment possible.

    B. Keeping you as comfortable as possible.

    C. Working to reduce any negative effects that might come from your treatments.

2. To help you stay happy and mentally strong. To keep an eye out for signs of sadness or worry, and if needed, start treatment early.

3. To offer love and social support, too. Ensuring your spiritual and religious needs are respected and fulfilled is important.

Although no two teams will ever be the same, successful teams have the needed skills and work well together. Build your team as soon as possible since pancreatic cancer can suddenly become overwhelming.

It's really important to accept help when friends offer it. If someone tells you, "I'll do anything to help," but then doesn't do anything, their words don't really mean a lot. One special way to let them help is for them to send over a meal. This can make the day a lot easier for your family. Also, there are many other ways people can be helpful, like giving you a lift to or from your treatments. Better yet, to stay with you if your infusion takes hours.

Patient Advocate

Every great team has a leader. Start with picking someone who can stand up for what you need and deserve. This person, known as a patient advocate, is there to provide emotional support, help build a team of caregivers, and help in making a detailed care plan. The best person for this job is someone who can provide a lot of support, like a husband, wife, or adult child. If you don't have anyone like this, don't worry—there are experts you can hire for this job.

Your helper should be prepared to invest a lot of time and be really involved. It's wise to pick someone who remains calm and knows your preferences, family situation, financial status, and other important things. They should also be ready to learn about complex medical information, different treatment options for your illness, and how insurance operates.

Choosing this person soon is important. Trust your instincts to help make your choice. Don't get too caught up in the details. You don't need to tell everyone whom you've picked as your patient advocate. This is to avoid any arguments or hurt feelings, especially if your family is already finding it hard to cope with your diagnosis. Instead, have one person who can accompany you to most of your doctor's visits. You'll rely heavily on this person for advice when making decisions about your treatment.

Overall, your care team's roles and tasks can be divided into three categories:

1. Emotional support

2. Information management

3. Medical care

Emotional Support Team

Your emotional support team is like your personal cheerleading squad. It is made up of your family, old friends, new friends and paid professionals. Your mix will depend on your preferences, how close (emotionally and geographically) your family is and your financial resources. Start by getting this group together at the beginning of your two-week "pause" period.

If you have more money, you might hire more helpers to take care of you at home. If you have less money, you'll probably rely on family and friends to help you out instead. But remember, *money makes you wealthy, but friends make you rich.*

You might be surprised to find out that people you aren't very familiar with, like your neighbors a few houses down or coworkers you do not work with directly, will also want to help you. They may offer things like airline miles, hotel points, or restaurant gift cards. If they do, don't turn them down. Instead, just say thank you. Remember, we're social beings, and absorbing all the positive energy can truly make a difference.

Information Management Team

Treating pancreatic cancer involves a lot of information. Often, a family member or a good friend is really good at organizing. This person would be perfect for the job. This job includes two main tasks: managing medical information and taking care of financial matters and insurance details. One person could do both parts or two could divide the work.

Medical Care Team

First, get the right family and friends together to form a medical care team. Then, you work together to pick doctors who know a lot about cancer and other doctors to help with related issues as listed below.

You may think looking at doctor ratings online is helpful but be careful! These ratings often do not tell the full story.[55] Sometimes, the websites do not check if the patient really met with the doctor they are rating. Plus, people who had a disappointing doctor's visit might make their experience seem worse than it was. This does not really show how good a doctor is. Also, reputation management companies can make doctors with bad reviews look good. So, do not believe everything you read in these online reviews![56]

1. *Oncologist* (covered by insurance):

An oncologist is a type of doctor who has extra training beyond medical school to become a specialist in cancer care. Just like how you keep studying to go to the next grade, these doctors study more after completing a residency in internal medicine to learn everything they can about cancer.

Imagine you're in school, learning different subjects like math, science, and English. Doctors are the same. After finishing medical school, some doctors decide to focus on one "subject" or area, like how you might prefer math or English. An oncologist is a doctor who decided to focus on

---

55. Ellimoottil, C., et al. (2013, September 1). Online physician reviews: The good, the bad, and the ugly. *Bulletin of the American College of Surgeons, 90*(9). Retrieved November 1, 2016, from http://bulletin.facs.org/2013/09/online-physician-reviews/

56. Glover, L. (2014, December 19). Are online physician ratings any good? *U.S. News and World Report.* http://health.usnews.com/health-news/patient-advice/articles/2014/12/19/are-online-physician-ratings-any-good

cancer as their main subject. They learn about how cancer starts, how it affects the body, and most importantly, how to fight it with different treatments. This extra studying makes them experts who can help people battling cancer in the best way possible.[57]

Oncologists are doctors who are really good at providing chemotherapy treatment, often shortened to "chemo." They know the right amount to give, how many days in a row to give it, and what side effects to look out for. They make changes if side effects occur. They make sure the nurses who give the treatment are safe in handling it and that the medicine is stored properly and given properly.

2. *Primary Care Physician* (covered by insurance):

Your main doctor, whom you usually see for check-ups and medical problems. They will work together with your oncologist to help you handle the problems from pancreatic cancer and from the treatments for it.

Chemotherapy can make you more likely to get infections. This is because it weakens your immune system, which normally helps you fight off sickness. If you get an infection and don't get help, it can lead to serious problems that might mean you need to go to the hospital immediately.

---

57. OpenAI. (2023). ChatGPT [Computer software]. Retrieved from https://www.openai.com/

Your primary care physician (PCP) works with your oncologist to take care of any new health problems that might come up because of the treatment for cancer. They try hard to keep these problems from getting really serious. As mentioned before, people with pancreatic cancer can get diabetes. If this happens, your PCP will treat it with medications.

People who get pancreatic cancer are an average of seventy years old[58] and often have other health problems. So, they also need their doctor to help them manage these other health issues. Your PCP will keep taking care of your other health problems, which might include things like high blood pressure or problems with your thyroid.

3. *Hepatobiliary Surgeon* (covered by insurance):

These doctors are experts in removing pancreatic cancers, making them highly respected in the world of medicine. After finishing medical school, they study and practice for another five years in hospitals. This time is called "surgical residency," and it's a super-long and important practice session. During this time, they work closely with expert surgeons who have been doing this for many years, learning how to become surgeons themselves. They get to try many types of surgeries and decide which ones they like best.

After finishing their residency, these doctors can decide

---

58. American Cancer Society. (2020, June 9). Pancreatic cancer risk factors. https://www.cancer.org/cancer/types/pancreatic-cancer/causes-risks-prevention/risk-factors.html

to do an extra training program called a "fellowship." This involves two more years of training that concentrate on surgeries related to one specific area of medicine or part of the body. A fellowship lets them learn more and get lots of practice in the surgery they most want to do. This helps them become top-notch experts in that surgery.

If a doctor wants to become a pro at doing surgeries on people with pancreatic cancer, they can choose from two types of fellowships. Both are good, but your doctor should have finished one of them. Remember to ask!

Hepatopancreatobiliary (HPB) Surgery Fellowship: This is a two-year program where a surgeon learns about liver, pancreas, and biliary tract diseases. You also get a lot of practice with complicated surgeries like the Whipple procedure (which will be described later).

Surgical Oncology Fellowship: Also, a two-year fellowship gives a surgeon the chance to become really good at the Whipple procedure, too. This is especially true in programs where there are many patients with pancreatic cancer.[59]

4. *Consulting Pathologist ($)*:

A pathologist is the kind of doctor who looks at cells, from a test called a biopsy. They look at these cells under

---

[59]. OpenAI. (2023). ChatGPT [Computer software]. Retrieved from https://www.openai.com/

a microscope. They use special methods such as chemical stains (dyes) to find out if the cells are healthy or if they have cancer. The first pathologist to look at your slides is usually a hospital employee who deals with all types of pathology—not a pathologist who specializes in pancreatic cancer.

When dealing with pancreatic cancer, it's really important to make sure you have the right diagnosis. This means knowing the exact kind of cancer you have. So, getting a second opinion from a consulting pathologist is a great idea. They can look at your biopsy slides (or pictures) again. This can be done at a place that specializes in pancreatic cancer, like a university hospital. Getting a second opinion might cost extra money. You can look up "pathology second opinion" online to find more details.

5. *Consulting Oncologist* **(often covered by insurance—$$ for travel):**

It's really smart to get a second opinion when you're dealing with pancreatic cancer. This means you should ask another cancer doctor who doesn't work with your current doctor, not even at the same hospital, what they think about your situation. This can help you make the best decisions about your treatment.

The doctors you seek for a second opinion should be academic oncologists. This means they are professors of medicine at medical schools. They will confirm the specific type and subtype of pancreatic cancer you have and give you different options for treatment. Or they might agree with your local doctor. This is valuable, too, because it gives you confidence in your local doctor.

It's important to know that the quality of cancer care and the way doctors approach treatment can vary between different hospitals and doctors. This can be surprising and worrying, so getting a second opinion can help you make more informed decisions about your care.

6. *Consulting Radiologist* ($$):

A radiologist is a type of doctor who looks at pictures of your body to see if your cancer is growing or spreading. These pictures can be taken using different kinds of imaging techniques, such as special types of X-rays, CT scans, MRI scans, and ultrasounds. There are special types of each for specific purposes. The radiologist will write a report about how many tumors you have and the size and shape of each. By studying the pictures, the radiologist can also tell if your tumor is near any important blood vessels or if it's blocking tubes like the bile or pancreatic duct.

Some radiologists have lots of experience with pancreatic cancer and may see things other radiologists do not. You may want an expert to look at your pictures, doing what is called an "overread," a second opinion by an expert radiologist. You can send your medical images on a CD, which might involve a small fee. To find more information, you can go online and search for "pancreatic cancer radiology second opinion."

7. *Concierge Primary Care Doctor* ($$$-$$$+):

A special type of primary care doctor is known as a concierge doctor. From AI: "Concierge medicine is a type of healthcare where you pay a monthly or yearly fee. This fee allows you to have quick and personal access to a doctor whenever you need it."[60] A concierge doctor and their staff can be very helpful if you have pancreatic cancer. They can assist you in finding other doctors to consult with and suggest various options to research for treating your cancer.

Additionally, they can help coordinate the efforts of all the other doctors and others involved in your care. They can arrange any necessary tests and guide you in navigating health insurance. Some even make house calls.

If you discover that you have pancreatic cancer, it's important to talk promptly to your regular doctor to determine how much they can support your treatment and consider a concierge primary care doctor.

---

60. OpenAI. (2023). ChatGPT [Computer software]. Retrieved from https://www.openai.com/

8. *Palliative Care Physician* (often covered by insurance):

Doctors who focus on a special area called hospice and palliative medicine do things a little differently. Their main goal is to help lessen symptoms like pain, upset stomach, nausea, night sweats, and other issues. They also assist you in feeling hungry again.

9. *Home nursing/Home Health Care* (Ranging from $$-$$$$)—AI assisted information:

Nurses are very helpful to those who can afford their services. Nowadays, more people are getting medical care at home, leading to shorter stays in the hospital or even avoiding hospital stays entirely. This is a big change from how it was twenty years ago.

There can be many uncomfortable symptoms from pancreatic cancer and its treatment. Many people prefer having a home health professional to help with issues related to bodily fluids rather than relying on a family member.

A. *Registered Nurse (RN)* ($$$$):

Education: Nursing education varies in length: an Associate Degree in Nursing (ADN) typically takes 2 years and is focused on basic nursing skills, while a Bachelor of

Science in Nursing (BSN) requires about 4 years, offering a more comprehensive education. Both pathways prepare students specifically to become Registered Nurses (RNs) by qualifying them for the NCLEX-RN exam. "Nursing school" can refer to either type of program, hence the 2 to 4-year range in study duration.

In the field of home nursing, RNs care for patients in the patients' homes, following the instructions and advice of doctors. Usually, doctors meet patients in their offices and not in the patients' homes. They rely on the nurses' notes to understand the patient's condition and provide further guidance. Only certain doctors, like those in concierge medicine or hospice care, regularly visit patients at home. This means that the quality of home nursing greatly depends on the RN's abilities and skills. Home nursing allows for personalized care of each patient, adapting to their unique needs.

Skills: Registered nurses need to be really good at looking after patients, making decisions, and talking clearly with patients and doctors. They also must know a lot about health and medicine. A key part of their job is to give patients their prescribed medicines and keep track of these medications. RNs also need to be able to handle emergencies and work well with other health care team members

B. Licensed Practical Nurse (LPN) or Licensed Vocational Nurse (LVN) (the title used in California and Texas) ($$$+):

Education: After they finish high school or an equivalent program, they attend school for at least one year. Once they complete their schooling, they take a test to get a special nursing license from the state. LPNs work with doctors or RNs and follow their instructions.

Skills: LPNs and LVNs have important jobs in healthcare. They follow instructions from doctors and RNs, take care of patients, and do basic medical tasks. Some of their duties include recording patients' vital signs like blood pressure, temperature, and pulse. They also report on the patient's condition to RNs and doctors, and add this information to the patient's charts. Additionally, they change wound dressings, give certain medications, and help with feeding and bathing patients.

C. Certified Nursing Assistants ($$+):

Education: They go through at least six weeks of special training. After that, they take and pass a test to get certified. They're not officially called nurses, but they play a big role in taking care of patients. Often, they work at night, helping in many ways.

Skills: Certified Nursing Assistants are skilled in measuring vital signs like temperature and blood pressure. They carefully watch patients for any important changes in their health. They help patients move around safely to prevent falls and keep them clean and comfortable. CNAs also assist with daily activities like eating and dressing, and ensure the patient's environment is safe and hygienic.

D. *Home Health Aide (HHA)/Nursing Assistants* ($$):

Education: Home Health Aides, unlike CNAs, may not always go through the same kind of formal training or state-required tests. **Some** of them learn a lot from their experience working with patients. While they do help with daily tasks and care, it's important to know that their training and experience can vary.

Skills: Home health aides need to be very caring and pay close attention to their patients. They help with daily tasks like bathing, dressing, and eating. It's also important for them to be good at listening and communicating, as they often need to understand and respond to the needs of their patients. Besides, they might also do some light cleaning and help patients remember when to take their medicines. But, it's important for patients be able to take their own medications because home health aides aren't trained or allowed to give out medicine.

E. Physical Therapist (PT)—AI Assisted:

Education: To become a Physical Therapist (PT), one must earn a Doctor of Physical Therapy degree, which usually requires about 7 years of college education. After completing the degree, passing a licensing exam is necessary to practice as a PT.

Skills: Physical Therapists need to work well in teams, show compassion, demonstrate leadership, and pay close attention to details. They should be skilled at teaching patients different exercises and have a good understanding of how the body moves. Being physically strong can also be helpful, as they often need to lift or assist patients in moving.

F. Physical Therapist Assistant (PTA)—AI Assisted:

Education: To become a Physical Therapist Assistant (PTA), you need an Associate Degree, which you can earn in two years. After finishing your degree, you must pass a state exam to get licensed to work.

Skills: PTAs must follow the treatment plans created by physical therapists to help patients. They need to be physically strong because they often help move patients and handle various equipment.[61]

---

61. OpenAI. (2023). ChatGPT [Computer software]. Retrieved from https://www.openai.com/

G. Occupational Therapist (OT):

Education: Occupational Therapists (OTs) need to get a master's or doctoral degree in occupational therapy. After finishing their degree, they have to pass a national exam to receive their license to practice.

Skills: OTs assist patients with their daily activities, which requires them to be excellent at solving problems and thinking creatively. They also need to be patient and good at explaining things clearly to help patients understand and perform various activities.

H. Speech Language Pathologist (SLP):

Education: Speech-Language Pathologists (SLPs) need to earn a master's degree in Speech-Language Pathology which includes many hours of working with patients under supervision. After completing their degree, they must pass a national exam to get their professional license.

Skills: SLPs work with patients who have speech and language difficulties. Therefore, they need to be very good at listening and speaking. Being patient and supportive is also important, as they help people improve their communication abilities.[62]

---

62. OpenAI. (2023). ChatGPT [Computer software]. Retrieved from https://www.openai.com/

10. ***Psychiatrists and Psychologists*** (sometimes covered by insurance, otherwise, ranging from $ to $$$):

>Just because you have pancreatic cancer, it does not mean you have to be depressed or in emotional distress.[63] Even those who do not tend to be depressed or anxious can easily become so. Talking with a mental health expert can help you manage their feelings better. This can include getting medication for anxiety, sleep problems, and depression. These experts can offer support and guidance on how to cope with these challenges.

>Psychologists and psychiatrists play different roles in mental health care, but both are essential. Psychiatrists are medical doctors with medical school training and a residency in psychiatry. They can prescribe medications and often focus on how these can help with mental health issues. Psychiatrists can also offer counselling (talk therapy).

>Psychologists typically hold a doctoral degree in psychology, such as a PhD or PsyD, and may also have a master's degree in a related field. However, unlike psychiatrists, they are not medical doctors. They spend more time talking and building a relationship with patients, using methods like Cognitive Behavioral Therapy. This rapport is key; if you don't feel connected with your psychologist or psychiatrist, it's okay to look for another one who suits you better.

---

63. National Cancer Institute. (2023, April 12). Adjustment to cancer: Anxiety and distress (PDQ®).https://www.cancer.gov/about-cancer/coping/feelings/anxiety-distress-hp-pdq

For some people, seeing a counselor with a master's degree might be perfect and less expensive. They can provide valuable support, especially for less complex mental health issues or general emotional support. They're also a part of the team helping with mental health, alongside psychologists and psychiatrists. Remember, finding the right mental health professional is an important part of your care, especially when dealing with challenging situations like pancreatic cancer.

Even though friends and family can listen and try to help, mental health experts have special skills that make them really good at helping. First, they've been trained to listen in a certain way, ask the right questions, and give useful advice. Second, since it's their job to help and they're getting paid for it, you don't have to worry about bothering them.

Sadly, many people with pancreatic cancer who should get help from talking to a mental health expert don't choose to do so. It's a good idea to reach out to a mental health expert if you need support.

11. *Interventional Radiologist* **(usually covered by insurance):**

Interventional radiologists do liver biopsies, which are minimally invasive and can be done through the skin or the jugular vein. Don't worry, this procedure is safe, and complications are rare. They also perform a procedure called Y-90, discussed in Step Ten. The cost of these consultations and procedures can vary depending on your insurance coverage.

12. *Oncology Nurses* (covered by insurance):

The oncology nurses are the ones who give you your chemotherapy through an IV. You don't get to choose them since they work at the chemotherapy treatment centers. But they play a crucial role in your team of caregivers. IV chemotherapy is like giving your body a small amount of poison to fight cancer. That's why nurses need to be very careful, both for your safety and their own. Some chemotherapy drugs can be harmful if inhaled or touched by the nurse.

13. *Genetic Counselor* (often covered by insurance):

Genetic counselors are specialists who provide guidance on genetic testing, particularly important for pancreatic cancer patients. They can assess whether there's cancer risk genes and evaluate the risk for family members.

Talking to a genetic counselor early on, when you're first diagnosed, can be really important. This step can improve how well treatment works for some people. But, it's key for patients to understand that their health insurance might not pay for everything. Some insurance plans might help pay for a basic meeting with a genetic counselor, but they may not cover the more detailed genetic tests.

This approach could significantly improve treatment strategies. However, it's important for patients to know that insurance coverage for genetic counseling can differ, with some plans covering basic consultations but not in-depth genetic evaluations.

14. *Biochemist* (no cost if you are in a clinical trial):

A biochemist specializing in pancreatic cancer studies this specific disease and typically holds a high-level degree like a Ph.D. Their work is focused on uncovering new insights about pancreatic cancer and dealing with complex scientific concepts. These professionals are involved in growing pancreatic organoids in special labs. They also conduct high-throughput testing. Another area they study is the potential of comparing a patient's DNA with their tumor's genetic profile. Especially with the aid of AI analysis, this is an exciting development in personalized medicine.

While biochemists might suggest innovative treatment approaches based on their research, they generally do not provide direct patient care, unless they are also qualified as medical doctors (M.D. or D.O.). Consulting with a biochemist can be very expensive ($$$+), except if you are part of a clinical trial, where there might be no cost involved.

Step Three: Get Organized

Staying organized is very important. When you're not feeling your best, this can be tough to do on your own. So, letting your teammates help you stay organized is a good idea.

Sometimes, a single piece of information can be essential. Other times, seeing a pattern on a chart can help decide treatment. Set up a system that works for you depending on how good you are with computers. It can be anything from using high-tech tools to just using three-ring binders.

We often say we are a "paperless" society. Still, oddly enough, we are dealing with more paper now than we ever did. You should take all your documents, like lab results, medical records, and insurance statements, and scan them into your computer. If you give these scanned files clear names and keep them organized, finding and using them when needed will be much easier. Keeping the actual paper documents for at least two years is a good idea. You could regret throwing them away or shredding them too soon.

It is essential to have a medical summary sheet (MSS) that has all your recent medical information. You should always keep it so you have it if you need emergency medical help. Having multiple copies in a folder is a good idea so you can hand it out whenever you go to the doctor or hospital. It might be helpful to have the information on a flash drive, too. However, many hospitals and doctors won't use it because they worry about computer viruses/digital security.

The Medical Summary Sheet (MSS) is also handy for regular doctor check-ups and cancer treatment sessions. Besides your photo ID and insurance card(s), the health care team will want to know these basic things (list assisted by AI):

1. Your name, phone number, insurance details, social security number, and birth date.

2. The kind of pancreatic cancer you have (like adenocarcinoma) and if it has spread to other parts of your body.

3. Any other health problems you have (like diabetes and high blood pressure).

4. Any past surgeries you have had.

5. The medicines you are taking now, including how much (usually in milligrams) and how many times a day you take them.

6. Your latest lab test and imaging results.

7. CD(s) of your most recent CT scan(s).

8. If you are allergic to any medicines, what kind of reaction you had, and when it happened.

9. Your history with smoking and drinking: Have you ever smoked? If so, for how long? How many packs per day? If you stopped, when? How many drinks do you have in an average day? Average week? If you were a heavy drinker and stopped, detail that also. It is essential to be honest because this information can help your doctor give you the best care.

10. The name and phone number of your primary doctor and oncologist.

11. Code status: If you become very sick, do you want to be revived using strong measures like electric shocks or a breathing tube? If you choose "do not resuscitate," you must tell the emergency room team unless you have a legal paper saying this.[64]

12. Whether you have a medical power of attorney or a health care surrogate and a copy of it if you do.

Keeping more detailed information than just what is in the MSS is important. Whether you rely on your computer, a combination of computer and paper, or only a paper system, you will need three main categories to organize your information:

---

64. OpenAI. (2023). ChatGPT [Computer software]. Retrieved from https://www.openai.com/

1. Symptoms before diagnosis: Write down any symptoms you experienced before your diagnosis.

2. Date of diagnosis: Record the exact date you were diagnosed with your condition.

3. History of your treatment(s): This section should include the following:

    A. Visits to the oncologist: Summarize what was discussed and decided during each visit, organized by date.

    B. Dates and types of all treatments: List the dates and any treatments you have undergone.

    C. Side effects: Note any side effects you have experienced, and the medicine you thought caused them.

    D. Imaging dates and reports: Include the dates of any imaging tests, such as x-rays and CT scans. Keep copies of the reports and the physical discs. You can use plastic CD holders designed for three-ring binders to store the CDs of your CT scans. If possible, request three CDs for each scan—one for yourself and two extras to give to specialists in the future. Additional CDs should be free or available at a minimal cost.

    E. Lab reports: Keep all your lab reports and other medical tests you have taken in order, starting with the newest first. If something urgent happens, like getting a fever on a Saturday night, having these reports with you when you go to the emergency room can be helpful. The hospital could get your test results directly in a perfect world, but this does not always happen. The emergency department can repeat some basic tests but not the cancer specific ones.

Your health insurance will likely swamp you with many confusing papers called "explanation of benefits" and other financial papers from your doctors. If you have been to a hospital, it can be even more puzzling. Hospitals often send out more papers than doctors' offices, and sometimes you might receive two or even three copies of the same thing in the mail. Here's how to handle all these papers:

1. After you look over the papers, keep them all in one place. You could use a big binder with rings to hold them, but a cardboard box with labeled folders will also work.

2. Put your papers in order by the date of your medical care, not by the date on the bill.

3. Use a paper clip to hold together papers that look the same, but don't throw anything away for at least a couple of years.

Creating, storing, and updating this information is a time-consuming job. If you are in the $$ category or above, I suggest offering at least some compensation to the friend, adult child, or adult grandchild who helps you. The task requires organizational and computer skills and enough discipline to update daily or at least several times a week. For those in the $$$ and $$$$ categories, some professionals and companies offer patient advocacy, data management, and health-bill-review services.

Likewise, there is often someone in your close circle who is a whiz at research whom we'll call an information finder. The internet and social media give us a lot of information, but it can be hard to check if it's true or not. It's a good idea to read newspaper articles, magazine articles, and books, which you can find through internet searches and on social media. I further recommend videos to help you understand the biology of the pancreas and pancreatic cancer treatment. The American Cancer Society has a pancreatic cancer treatment summary page.[65]

The latest and most reliable news often appears first in medical journals (science magazines), and newspapers also report it. These articles about health and science topics are usually accurate and easy to find. Plus, you can often find short summaries of science articles for free online. For full articles, I suggest reading just the beginning and end parts (abstract and conclusion) of these science articles. The middle part is usually long and has unfamiliar words that might not really help you with your health issues. Based on what you and your team learn, make a list of questions and topics to discuss with your cancer doctor.

Finally, it's all right to change things up if someone on your team isn't doing a good job. Maybe you can find a different job for them and get someone else to do what they were doing before.

---

65. American Cancer Society. (2023). Treating pancreatic cancer. Retrieved from https://www.cancer.org/cancer/types/pancreatic-cancer/treating.html

Step Four: Choose Your Oncologist

Picking the right cancer doctor or oncologist is a very important choice. You should use a mix of doing your homework, common sense, and listening to your gut feeling. Remember, oncologists are special doctors who know how to find and treat cancer. Choosing the right one for you can make your treatment much better. This chapter will help you make that choice easier.

This summarizes how oncologists become certified experts:

1. They graduate from college—usually four years of study.

2. They go to medical school for another four years.

3. New doctors aiming to become oncologists usually spend three years in a program for internal medicine. During this time, they take care of patients and are supervised by more experienced doctors.

4. Then they do a fellowship for two to three more years, where they learn all about treating cancer.

The American Board of Internal Medicine has a website you can use to see if the oncologist you're thinking about choosing is board-certified. Being board-certified means they've passed important tests and meet certain standards, so you know they're well-trained.[66] The exception is some oncologists are very well trained, often in Europe, but not eligible for US board certification.

You should also look up where they went to medical school, where they did their residency, and where they had their fellowship. It's a good idea to see if they did their fellowship at a well-known medical school that gets high rankings from *U.S. News & World Report*. This can help you feel more confident that they're a good choice.[67]

However, education is only part of what you should consider. You should also verify the doctor's medical license (see Appendix A for how to do this), ensuring it's valid and in effect. If it isn't easy to find, there might be simple explanations, such as a recent name or address change due to marriage. More importantly, check for any state board of medicine sanctions or "public complaints." These are rare and would be important to know about.

---

66. ABIM. (n.d.). Important information regarding the physician verification tool. Retrieved July 12, 2023, from https://www.abim.org/verify-physician

67. Chau, Z., West, J. K., Zhou, Z., McDade, T., Smith, J. K., Ng, S. C., Kent, T. S., Callery, M. P., Moser, A. J., & Tseng, J. F. (2014). Rankings versus reality in pancreatic cancer surgery: a real-world comparison. *HPB: the official journal of the International Hepato Pancreato Biliary Association*, *16*(6), 528-533. https://doi.org/10.1111/hpb.12171

When you meet different cancer doctors, notice how they talk to you. Do they really listen and answer your questions? Or do they make you feel rushed? How you feel about them can tell you a lot about how they treat their patients.

Usually, doctors decide what to do based on how advanced the cancer is and the patient's overall health. Sometimes, removing the cancer through surgery is possible, but often it's not. That's when chemotherapy might be used.

Some people worry that doctors could be influenced by making extra money by giving chemotherapy in their infusion centers. However, there are rules and guidelines to help make sure that doctors suggest the best treatment for their patients. If you are worried about this, it's a good idea to get a second opinion from another doctor to make sure the treatment plan is best for you.

The cancer doctor you pick should be ready and happy to work with other doctors and health experts. They should get along well with a team of doctors who have different specialties. They should also be willing to talk about your treatment with this team. It's okay if they email, but it's even better if they can have a group phone call about once a month, even if not everyone can join in each time.

If you're thinking about trying other kinds of treatments, like alternative therapies, insurance might need to approve it first. Your oncologist should help you with this and try to get your approval.[68]

---

68. Cancer.Net. (2023, February 10). Pancreatic Cancer—Types of Treatment. https://www.cancer.net/cancer-types/pancreatic-cancer/types-treatment

If you mostly speak a language other than English, it's good to know that you usually have the right to get a medical interpreter. This is the law in many states. The interpreter can talk with you on the phone or online. You usually don't have to pay for it; the doctor's office often covers the cost. It's very important to use a medical interpreter when you first meet the doctor or have other big appointments.

You might think that asking a family member to help you understand the doctor is a good idea. But medical words can be hard to translate into another language. Also, a family member might not tell you exactly what the doctor said because they want to protect your feelings or influence your choices. That's why it's a good idea to use a professional medical interpreter to make sure you understand everything clearly.

There are laws that ensure everyone gets fair treatment at the doctor's office. These laws also assist people who have trouble seeing or hearing. Here are some of the laws that do this:

- Title VI of the Human Rights Act

- Medicare Access & CHIP Reauthorization Act of 2015

- Section 1557 of the Affordable Care Act

These laws make sure you get the right care, no matter what language you speak or what challenges you have.

Steps Five, Six and Seven: Pathology, Radiology and Oncology Second Opinions

(Start asking for appointments at the same time —get in any order)

Just like laying a solid foundation is essential before building a house, it's crucial to be sure you have pancreatic cancer, identify the specific type, and determine if it has spread before beginning any treatment. I suggest getting another doctor to look at your pathology slides and imaging, like CT scans, to give a second opinion. Again, this is called "overreading" in this situation.

It's a bit better to have your pathology and radiology second opinion/expert reports before you get a second pancreatic cancer doctor's expert opinion about your cancer. But don't worry if you don't have the pathology and radiology overreads yet. The doctor can look at them later. Start to get all these expert opinions at the same time. Time matters a lot, and making appointments can be frustrating and time-consuming.

Get a Pathology Second Opinion

A pathology slide is like a thin sheet with a person's cells placed on a glass. To help see them better under a microscope, special chemicals are used to color the cells. These slides can also be turned into digital images (pictures on a computer) for analysis. The doctors who study and analyze these slides are pathologists. They have a very important job in diagnosing different illnesses. Pathologists also give the final and definite diagnosis of pancreatic cancer, while radiologists figure out if it has spread to other places in the body.[69]

Pathologists also study samples of body tissue to identify the kind of pancreatic cancer a person has. The most common type is adenocarcinoma. In a group of 100 people with pancreatic cancer, about 95 would have this type. The other 5 might have something different, like neuroendocrine tumors. Steve Jobs had this less common type[70]

Pathologists do more than just identify the cancer type. They also find out other important information, like how fast the cancer cells are growing. Then, they share this information with your oncologist who needs to know the details about your cancer cells to determine the best treatment for you. That could be surgery, chemotherapy, or other methods. So, the patholo-

---

69. American Cancer Society. (2019, February 11). What is pancreatic cancer?: Types of pancreatic cancer.https://www.cancer.org/cancer/types/pancreatic-cancer/about/what-is-pancreatic-cancer.html
70. Harmon, K. (2011, October 7). The puzzle of pancreatic cancer: How Steve Jobs did not beat the odds—but Nobel winner Ralph Steinman did. *Scientific American* https://www.scientificamerican.com/article/pancreatic-cancer-type-jobs/

gist and the oncologist work together like a team to help the patient get the best treatment possible.

You can find a special hospital, known as an academic medical center, to send your biopsy slides. Just search "pathology second opinion" on the internet to find options. A second look at your disease sample usually costs about $250 ($). The price might go up if more tests are needed. Your insurance may not cover this cost. Even if money is tight, getting a second opinion on your pathology slides is a smart move.

Your first pathologist will usually be correct, but it is very important to catch any mistakes early on. Even discovering a slight change in your kind of pancreatic cancer can help you get better treatment.

Get an Oncology Second Opinion(s)

I am repeating this quote from the Hope chapter because it fits so well in both places:

> Although the chemo that was recommended was the same chemo my health care provider in California recommended, MSK [Memorial Sloan Kettering Cancer Center, New York, NY] had done a recent clinical trial in which they found the chemo was as effective at 85% as it was at 100%. The issue was that particular chemo at 100% was so toxic that most people couldn't tolerate it. I believe that I'm alive today because of that visit. **JG**

I have had many patients who have been hesitant to travel to for medical care with excuses of cost and inconvenience, especially to their family. Yet these same people go on business trips, weekend trips for sports, entertainment, and vacations. A trip to see a specialist is not much different than these trips (although not as fun) but is often much more valuable. If you haven't already read, "Why a Top Cancer Center Could Save Your Life,"[71] read it now!

Let's talk about two kinds of doctors who help people with cancer. The first one is a general cancer doctor, also known as an oncologist. The second one is an oncologist who only treats pancreatic cancer.

The general cancer doctor is usually closer to your home and may be able to give you more personal care. But the doctor specializing in pancreatic cancer knows a lot more about this type of cancer. They are professors of medicine at medical schools and academic medical centers. They know about and are doing the latest research and treatments for pancreatic cancer.

Either the general oncologist or the expert cancer doctor can be the first one you see for cancer. Often, your PCP diagnoses your cancer and sends you to a local cancer doctor they know. I strongly recommend that you see a doctor specializing in pancreatic cancer before you begin treatment. They can ensure that you're diagnosed right and recommend the best treatment to start with.

---

71. Begley, S. (2009, October 16). Why a top cancer center could save your life. *Newsweek*. http://www.newsweek.com/why-top-cancer-center-could-save-your-life-81425

If you can't have surgery, you can be treated closer to home by the general cancer doctor. You should talk to the office staffs to make sure your medical records are sent from your local doctor **and received** by the expert at the academic center. This keeps the expert informed and ready to help during treatment.

Don't forget, it's up to you to choose your cancer doctor(s). Trust your gut, get advice from your team, and think clearly when making your choice. You want a doctor who will be there to support you as you work to get better.

Even the smartest experts don't have all the answers, especially when it comes to complex issues like pancreatic cancer. Treatments for this type of cancer are still developing and can have strong side effects. Because of this, exploring different options and getting advice from multiple sources may be helpful.

Meeting with doctors **in person** at top cancer hospitals can be more helpful for your care. They will examine you and talk to you in person. Your conversation with the expert is often the most important part because information is exchanged both ways. These doctors are experts in treating pancreatic cancer and other stomach-related cancers.

Your health insurance might pay for you to see a pancreatic cancer expert. Some do, some don't. Make sure to check your insurance before seeing the expert.

Before you talk to the second doctor, try to learn about new treatments. Look for ones that seem to work well. When you meet the expert and their medical team, ask them about these options.

Also, talk about your concerns, especially if you're worried that no treatment might be effective or worth taking. Ask how they would advise their family member facing similar challenges.

To keep track of these important topics, it's a good idea to make a brief list of your questions and concerns. Practicing what you want to say or ask will help you feel more confident and ensure you cover everything important during your discussion. This way, the doctor can give you more information and help you decide what's best for your situation.[72]

Getting an appointment with specialists can be hard, especially quickly. Here are some tips to help you book one:

- Find the direct phone number for the doctor's office.

- Try to avoid the central call center or the place where they set up all the appointments.

- Be polite and kind when you call.

- Share why you need the appointment urgently.

- Ask if they can contact you about cancellations so you can be seen earlier. Say that you are willing to come anytime, even on short notice.

---

72. Nita Ahuja and JoAnn Coleman, *Patients' Guide to Pancreatic Cancer* (Burlington, MA: Jones and Bartlett Learning, 2012), 35-37. Reprinted with permission.

Ask people you know for help. This could include family, friends, influential people, someone on the hospital's board of directors, a big donor to the hospital, or your doctor. For this disease, even friends of friends are often willing to help.

Here are some questions that AI suggests you could ask your doctor if you or a loved one has pancreatic cancer:

1. What kind and stage of pancreatic cancer do I have?

2. Would you explain my pathology report?

3. What treatment options are available for my cancer type and stage?

4. What are the pros and cons of these treatments?

5. Is surgery possible? What would it involve?

6. What's the goal of the treatment you suggest?

7. How will the treatment affect my daily life?

8. Can I still work, exercise, and do my usual activities?

9. What side effects might the treatment have, and how can we manage them?

10. Are there any clinical trials that might work for me?

11. Should I get another opinion?

12. What are the chances the cancer will come back after treatment?

13. What kind of care will I need after treatment?

14. Can you suggest any places where I can find more information or support?

15. Are there any diet changes I should make?

16. Should I see a genetic counselor?

AI adds:

Remember, everyone's situation is different. You might have other or additional questions, and the answers can depend on your specific case. Always ask your doctor anything you want to know, and make sure you understand their answers. If you're confused, don't be shy to ask them to explain again.[73]

If you can't travel to a big cancer center, there's another good option. Many cancer centers offer chart reviews, where they look at your medical records and even check your diagnostic images like X-rays, CT scans, and MRIs. This can change your treatment and your life. This service currently costs around

---

73. OpenAI. (2023). ChatGPT [Computer software]. Retrieved from https://www.openai.com/

$1,000 and may not be covered by your health insurance. To locate a doctor for this service, search "Telemedicine pancreatic cancer second opinion" online, or reach out to PanCAN Patient Services at 877-272-6226.[74]

Remember, when you talk to a second doctor for another opinion, ask about treatments that maybe your local oncologist did not mention. Your local oncologist is probably great, but they do not know everything. For example, a local cancer doctor might not tell you about a special kind of medicine for pancreatic cancer, the low-dose chemotherapy that **JG** told us about.

The cancer doctors near you will usually work well with you and your family. Plus, it's convenient because their office is close to your home. The best balance between local and cancer center care is up to you and depends on how bad your cancer is and what you prefer. Again, for emphasis, it's often good to have an expert doctor confirm your diagnosis and recommend the treatment to start with, then get that treatment from a nearby doctor.

Get a Radiology Second Opinion(s)

Pancreatic cancer can be tough to find and diagnose because it involves a complex part of our bodies. This is why if a doctor thinks you might have it, they'll use pictures like X-rays, ultrasounds, CT scans, and MRIs to get a closer look. But read-

---

74. Pancreatic Cancer Action Network. (2023, February 6). Considering a second opinion. *Pancreatic Cancer Action Network*. Retrieved from https://pancan.org/facing-pancreatic-cancer/diagnosis/choosing-your-healthcare-team/considering-a-second-opinion/

ing these images is like trying to solve a tricky puzzle—it takes a lot of knowledge and practice. Getting a second opinion from a radiologist at an academic medical center can really help.

An academic medical center is like a school for radiologists. Their senior doctors are always learning and teaching about the latest ways to take pictures of the body and find cancer. The radiologists at these places are very good at looking at these tricky images. They often know a lot about specific body parts, like the pancreas, and are always finding new ways to see issues.

Getting a second radiology opinion means you have another expert checking your images. This is important because sometimes even the best doctors can miss something or see things differently. A second look by a radiologist at an academic medical center can catch anything missed or confirm what was found. This means you and your doctors can be sure about your diagnosis and make the best plan to treat it. So, getting a second opinion is always a good idea if you're dealing with something as serious as pancreatic cancer ($).

You can get a second opinion about your radiology pictures from far away or by going to a cancer center. Usually, you don't see the radiologist. It's easier now because medical images are digital, not on film. Radiologists review your images and write down what they find. Some are even willing to show you your images on a video conference call, explain what they see, and answer your questions.

AI adds: Finding an academic radiologist to review your imaging studies can be an important step in your care. Here are some suggestions on how to proceed:

1. **Referral from Your Current Health Care Provider:** Often, your primary care doctor or oncologist can refer you to an academic radiologist. They may have connections with specialists in academic centers who are experienced in interpreting complex cases like pancreatic cancer.

2. **Research Academic Medical Centers:** Look for major academic medical centers or university hospitals that have departments specializing in gastrointestinal diseases and cancer. These institutions often have radiologists who are experts in interpreting imaging studies for specific conditions like pancreatic cancer.

3. **Contact Radiology Departments Directly:** Once you've identified a few academic medical centers, you can contact their radiology departments directly. Explain your situation and ask if they have specialists who can overread your imaging studies.

4. **Digital Transfer of Images:** Many hospitals and imaging centers now use digital systems for imaging studies. Instead of getting a CD, ask if your imaging center can transfer your images electronically to the academic center. This method is faster and reduces the risk of data loss or damage that can occur with physical media like CDs.

(From the author: Transferring electronically is not always an option so overnighting a CD is a good Plan B)

5. **Privacy and Consent:** Remember that transferring medical records and images requires your consent due to privacy laws. Ensure that you complete any necessary consent forms that allow your current imaging center to share your images with the academic radiologist.

6. **Insurance and Cost Considerations:** Check with your insurance provider about coverage for second opinions or overreads by specialists at academic centers. Sometimes, there might be additional costs involved, and it's best to know these details beforehand.

7. **Support Groups and Advocacy Organizations:** Support groups and advocacy organizations for pancreatic cancer can also be valuable resources. They often have information on how to find specialists and can offer advice based on the experiences of other patients.

Remember, it's essential to stay proactive and informed about your health care options, and seeking a second opinion or expert review of your imaging studies is a wise step in managing your treatment.[75]

---

75. OpenAI. (2023). ChatGPT [Computer software]. Retrieved from https://www.openai.com/

Step Eight: Surgery, If Possible

After another round of testing, the surgeon informed me that my tumor was unresectable, and my best bet was to go home and start treatment with my oncologist and see how long it could sustain me.

"... If this is what your mom is facing, then this is the place she needs to be, and this is the surgeon she needs to see." [said to KH's son] That place was M.D. Anderson in Houston, Texas, and the surgeon was Dr. Doug Evans. In hindsight, it all just seemed that I was experiencing one miracle after another. With such a downer from the Seattle appointment, we decided to take our "angel" up on his suggestion and went to Houston. He was able to get us an appointment with Dr. Evans within 48 hours and we took the "red eye" (first class I might add) and set off for Houston. It was a hard day of testing—and our best hope was for a possible clinical trial.

The next morning, I met with Dr. Evans and his PA, and it didn't quite turn out the way we expected. Dr. Evans came into the exam room and immediately I felt confidence exuded from him (confidence and not arrogance). He smiled at me and said, "It's a large tumor—5 centimeters—but it's resectable. I feel it's 90% odds of being able to take it out." That was pretty good odds for us.

... If I got through this challenge, I would give back in any way I could to help others. I've kept that commitment for the last 13 years. **KH**

"Surgery, if possible" is this book's three most important words. According to PanCAN, "Although 20 percent of pancreatic cancer patients may be eligible for surgery, data shows that up to half of those patients are told they are ineligible."[76] Duke University says, "Up to 30% of people with pancreatic cancer may benefit from Whipple surgery, a complex operation that, when combined with chemotherapy, is considered the most effective treatment for pancreatic cancer."[77]

If a person has pancreatic cancer that has not spread to other parts of the body, they might be able to have surgery to remove it. About 1 in 5 people who have this surgery can be com-

---

76. PanCAN. (2021, September 29). Choosing your health care team. *Pancreatic Cancer Action Network*. Retrieved from https://pancan.org/facing-pancreatic-cancer/diagnosis/choosing-your-healthcare-team/
77. Duke Health. (n.d.). Whipple surgery for pancreatic cancer. Retrieved July 10, 2023, https://www.dukehealth.org/blog/whipple-surgery-pancreatic-cancer

pletely cured of the cancer.[78] To be a candidate for surgery, you must be in good overall health. Also, the cancerous lump in your pancreas should not be too closely intertwined with important nerves or blood vessels that are close by (see photo in Basics About Your Pancreas and Pancreatic Cancer).

Types of Pancreatic Surgery

Doctors can treat pancreatic cancer in several ways, depending on how far it's advanced and where it is, the patient's overall health, and other details. Different kinds of surgeries can help:

- **Whipple procedure:** Whipple surgery is often the best choice for pancreatic cancer. In some cases, it can even cure the disease. This surgery is especially helpful for people whose cancer hasn't spread too far. It's a major surgery, but for the right candidates, it can either cure or significantly extend their life, making it worth the risks and recovery time.

    This surgery is usually done when the cancer tumor is in the beginning part of the pancreas. In the operation, the doctor removes the starting section of the pancreas, a piece of the small intestine, the gallbladder, and part of a tube called the bile duct. Sometimes, they also take out a part of the stomach and tiny structures called lymph nodes.

---

78. Pancreatic Cancer—StatPearls. *NCBI Bookshelf.* (n.d.). National Library of Medicine. Retrieved from https://www.ncbi.nlm.nih.gov/books/NBK518996/

Lymph nodes help our bodies fight germs, but the cancer can also spread to them. This surgery is mainly used to treat a type of pancreatic cancer called adenocarcinoma.

- **Distal pancreatectomy:** The doctor does this surgery when the cancer tumor is in the body or "tail," which is the end part of the pancreas. In this operation, they remove the tail and sometimes a part of the body of the pancreas. They might even take out the spleen, an organ that helps us fight off infections. This type of surgery treats a special kind of pancreatic cancer called neuroendocrine pancreatic cancer. Famous people like Steve Jobs and Maria Menounos had this kind of cancer.

- **Total pancreatectomy:** In this operation, the doctor takes out the entire pancreas, a piece of the small intestine, part of the stomach, a tube called the common bile duct, the gallbladder, the spleen, and some lymph nodes close by. Doctors usually avoid this surgery because it can cause permanent digestion problems and always leads to diabetes. This happens because, after the surgery, the body can't make insulin anymore.

- **Palliative surgery:** If the cancer has spread too far and can't be fully removed, doctors might still perform surgery to make the patient feel better or to stop other health issues. For instance, if the tumor is blocking the small intestine or a tube called the bile duct, they might do a bypass surgery to clear the way.

- **Minimally invasive surgeries:** Sometimes, doctors use special techniques like laparoscopic surgery, which uses small tools and a tiny camera, or robotic surgery, where a machine controlled by the doctor does the work. These methods use smaller cuts on the body, which can mean less pain and faster healing for the patient.

Every surgery comes with its risks and issues, so doctors take their time to decide the best one to use. Knowing that not everyone with pancreatic cancer can have surgery is also key. Treatments like chemotherapy and radiation therapy can sometimes be used before surgery to make it possible or easier, by shrinking the tumor. Also, they sometimes use these therapies after surgery or if surgery can't be done.[79]

Choosing a Surgeon and Hospital

Doctors sometimes suggest quick surgery for pancreatic cancer, especially when it's causing serious issues. But if you're not in a very bad health situation, it's really important for a group of medical experts to work together to figure out if surgery is the best choice. This team should include surgeons specializing in cancer, doctors who are experts in chemotherapy, and doctors skilled in radiation therapy which is using x-rays to shrink tumors. They should think about what's best for you, considering your health and what you want. You should also

---

79. OpenAI. (2023). ChatGPT [Computer software]. Retrieved from https://www.openai.com/

talk with your doctors about the pros and cons of having surgery so you can make the best choice.[80]

When picking a surgeon, there are several important things to think about:

Experience

Pick a surgeon who has done many surgeries, especially the type you need. Their experience is very important for your surgery. For instance, only 54 surgeons in the country do 12 or more Whipples per year which is considered the minimal number to be an expert.[81] The death rate in the first 30 days after the operation for the expert surgeons was 1.8% vs. 4.7% for the surgeons who did fewer than 12 Whipples per year.[82]

If you can get this surgery, that's good news! But remember, it's a big deal and pretty risky. Even in hospitals where they do this surgery a lot, between 2 to 4 out of every 100 people die within 30 days of surgery. So, choose a surgeon with a lot of

---

80. OpenAI. (2023). ChatGPT [Computer software]. Retrieved from https://www.openai.com/
81. Nathan, H., & Sonnenday, C. (2020, May 12). *Surgical volume improves patient outcomes—but should related procedures count?* Institute for Healthcare Policy & Innovation. https://ihpi.umich.edu/news/surgical-volume-improves-patient-outcomes-should-related-procedures-count
82. "Association of Surgeon Case Numbers of Pancreaticoduodenectomies vs Related Procedures with Patient Outcomes to Inform Volume-Based Credentialing. (2020). *JAMA Network Open.* https://doi.org/10.1001/jamanetworkopen.2020.3850

experience to have the best chance of success.[83, 84]

New surgeons might not be ready for really tough cases yet. They often do simpler surgeries to get more practice and build a good track record. Sometimes, these new doctors might say a certain surgery can't be done, but really, it means they can't do it. A more experienced surgeon could.

Older, more skilled surgeons usually handle harder cases, often with older or sicker patients. So, if your case is tough, you'll want someone who's been around the block a few times.

How do you find out about a doctor's history with a certain type of surgery? It can be hard because this info isn't always easy to get.

There are ways to get this information. The best way is to simply ask the doctor or their office. They should have this info, and many doctors are okay with telling their patients about how many successful operations they've had, how many had problems, and other important facts. Plus, you can ask them how

---

83. Pugalenthi, A., Protic, M., Gonen, M., Kingham, T. P., Angelica, M. I., DeMatteo, R. P., Fong, Y., Jarnagin, W. R., & Allen, P. J. (2016). Postoperative complications and overall survival after pancreaticoduodenectomy for pancreatic ductal adenocarcinoma. *Journal of Surgical Oncology, 113*(2), 188-193. https://doi.org/10.1002/jso.24125

84. Winter, J. M., Cameron, J. L., Campbell, K. A., Arnold, M. A., Chang, D. C., Coleman, J., Hodgin, M. B., Sauter, P. K., Hruban, R. H., Riall, T. S., Schulick, R. D., Choti, M. A., Lillemoe, K. D., & Yeo, C. J. (2006). 1423 pancreaticoduodenectomies for pancreatic cancer: A single-institution experience. *Journal of Gastrointestinal Surgery, 10*, 1199-1210. Discussion 1210-1211.

much experience they have with the exact operation you need.[85]

You can also look online for scientific articles and websites that talk about different surgeons and their experience. These can give you a better idea of who's really good at the specific surgery you need. So, do some research, and it'll help you make a smarter choice!

The data about the Whipple surgery showed that more experienced surgeons are better than those with less experience:

- Complications after surgery: 39% for experienced surgeons vs. 53% for less-experienced surgeons.

- Leakage from the pancreas after surgery: 10% for experienced surgeons vs. 20% for less-experienced surgeons.

- Blood loss during surgery: 1101 mL for experienced surgeons vs. 1918 mL for less-experienced surgeons.

- How long the surgery takes: 335 minutes for experienced surgeons vs. 458 minutes for less-experienced surgeons.[86]

---

85. Schmidt, C. M., Turrini, O., Parikh, P., House, M. G., Zyromski, N. J., Nakeeb, A., Howard, T. J., Pitt, H. A., & Lillemoe, K. D. (n.d.). Effect of hospital volume, surgeon experience, and surgeon volume on patient outcomes after pancreaticoduodenectomy: A single institution experience. *JAMA Network*. https://jamanetwork.com/journals/jamasurgery/fullarticle/406128

86. Schmidt, C. M., Turrini, O., Parikh, P., House, M. G., Zyromski, N. J., Nakeeb, A., Howard, T. J., Pitt, H. A., & Lillemoe, K. D. (n.d.). Effect of hospital volume, surgeon experience, and surgeon volume on patient outcomes after pancreaticoduodenectomy: A single institution experience. *JAMA Network*. https://jamanetwork.com/journals/jamasurgery/fullarticle/406128

Hospital Reputation

It's easy to think that only the surgeon matters when you need a big surgery like one for pancreatic cancer. But where your operation will happen is also important. Top-rated cancer hospitals should be on your list.

Pancreatic surgery is tough and special. It needs many medical experts working together. During surgery, there's a big team. The main doctor is the surgeon, but there are also people like:

- **Anesthesiologists:** They make sure you're asleep and safe during surgery.

- **Surgical nurses and doctors in training:** They assist the surgeon.

- **Radiologists:** They read (interpret) medical images before, after and even during surgery.

- **Pathologists:** During the surgery, they check the removed tumor to see if all the cancer has been removed.[87]

After surgery, there's another team:

- **ICU doctors and nurses:** They take care of you right after surgery.

---

87. Khalifa, M. A. (2007). Intraoperative assessment of the Whipple resection specimen. *Journal of Clinical Pathology, 60*(9), 975-980. https://doi.org/10.1136/jcp.2006.044834

- **Gastroenterologists:** They monitor and care for your stomach and intestines.

- **Physical Therapists:** They help you move and get active again. It's really important! Their knowledge helps you figure out the best pace and exercises for you.

- **Nutritionists:** They help with what you should eat.

Together, they all make sure you get the best care. Every person on a team has special knowledge that helps to get the job done and make the patient feel better. So, even though the surgeon's job is important, the rest of the health care team is just as important. They all play a crucial role in managing the challenges of pancreatic surgery.

In a study of eleven hospitals, where a total of 804 surgeries to remove parts of the pancreas took place, the number of these surgeries a hospital did was linked with how well the patients did afterward.[88] However, this wasn't the strongest predictor we found.

The strongest link was between a hospital's rank in the *US News & World Report* and how well patients did after their surgeries. Healthgrades ratings, which are another way to score hospitals, didn't match up as well with patient outcomes. In a surprising twist, hospitals with better ratings from *Consumer*

---

88. Ho, V., & Heslin, M. J. (2003). Effect of hospital volume and experience on in-hospital mortality for pancreaticoduodenectomy. *Annals of Surgery, 237*(4), 509-514. https://doi.org/10.1097/01.SLA.0000059981.13160.97

Reports had worse patient outcomes.[89] These are the top *US News & World Report* rankings:

1. **University of Texas MD Anderson Cancer Center:** University of Texas MD Anderson Cancer Center in Houston, TX, is nationally ranked in 7 adult and 1 pediatric specialty and rated high performing in 1 adult specialty and 5 procedures and conditions. It is a cancer facility. It is a teaching hospital.

2. **Memorial Sloan Kettering Cancer Center:** Memorial Sloan Kettering Cancer Center in New York, NY, is nationally ranked in 7 adult and 1 pediatric specialty and rated high performing in 1 adult specialty and 4 procedures and conditions. It is a cancer facility. It is a teaching hospital.

3. **Mayo Clinic:** Mayo Clinic in Rochester, MN, is ranked No. 1 on the Best Hospitals Honor Roll. It is nationally ranked in 14 adult and 10 pediatric specialties and rated high performing in 1 adult specialty and 20 procedures and conditions. It is a general medical and surgical facility. It is a teaching hospital.

4. **Dana-Farber Brigham Cancer Center:** Dana-Farber Cancer Institute in Boston, MA, is nationally ranked in 1 adult and 1 pediatric specialty and rated high performing in 4 adult procedures and conditions. It is a cancer facil-

---

89. Chau, Z., West, J. K., Zhou, Z., McDade, T., Smith, J. K., Ng, S. C., Kent, T. S., Callery, M. P., Moser, A. J., & Tseng, J. F. (2014). Rankings versus reality in pancreatic cancer surgery: A real-world comparison. *HPB (Oxford), 16*(6), 528-533. https://doi.org/10.1111/hpb.12171

ity. It is a teaching hospital. *U.S. News* includes Brigham and Women's Hospital in evaluating the performance of Dana-Farber Cancer Institute in Cancer, Colon Cancer Surgery and Lung Cancer Surgery and includes Boston Children's Hospital in evaluating the performance of Dana-Farber Cancer Institute in Pediatric Cancer.

5. **UCLA Medical Center:** UCLA Medical Center in Los Angeles, CA, is ranked No. 5 on the Best Hospitals Honor Roll. It is nationally ranked in 14 adult and 7 pediatric specialties and rated high performing in 17 adult procedures and conditions. It is a general medical and surgical facility. It is a teaching hospital.[90]

One big advantage of cancer centers is their pathology department.[91] AI summarizes…

When someone has pancreatic cancer, where they get care matters a lot. A big academic center that sees a lot of pancreatic cancer patients has some advantages over a smaller community hospital:

1. **Right Diagnosis:** Academic centers have pathologists who see these cases often. They're really good at telling if a lump is cancer or not.

---

90. US News & World Report. (2023). Best hospitals for cancer | Rankings & Ratings—US News Health. Retrieved from https://health.usnews.com/best-hospitals/rankings/cancer
91. Khalifa, M. A. (2007). Intraoperative assessment of the Whipple resection specimen. *Journal of Clinical Pathology, 60*(9), 975-980. https://doi.org/10.1136/jcp.2006.044834

2. **Staging:** These centers have advanced tools and experts who are used to figuring out how big the cancer is and if it has spread.

3. **Margins:** After surgery, pathologists at these centers are very detailed in checking if all the cancer has been removed.

4. **Special Tests:** They can do advanced tests that might not be available at smaller hospitals. This helps choose the best medicine.

5. **Teamwork:** In big centers, doctors often work together in teams focused on pancreatic cancer. They share their knowledge and make joint plans.

6. **Learning & Research:** Academic centers often do research and are up-to-date with the latest findings. This means patients can get the newest treatments.

7. **Quality Checks:** With many experts and strict standards, these centers ensure their work is top-notch.

In short, while all hospitals aim to provide good care, a high-volume academic center has special expertise in pancreatic cancer, making it a great choice for the best possible treatment.[92]

---

92. OpenAI. (2023). ChatGPT [Computer software]. Retrieved from https://www.openai.com/

If you need Whipple surgery, you should also consider the following:

1. Dr. Christopher Wolfgang

He is a surgeon at from NYU Langone Health in New York City and is very experienced. He has performed over 1,200 Whipple surgeries. Before NYU, he worked at Johns Hopkins.[93]

2. Duke Health (Durham, NC)

At Duke, more than 100 Whipple procedures are performed annually. "Combined, our surgeons have performed more than 1,500 Whipple procedures," said Peter Allen, MD, chief of surgical oncology, who specializes in pancreatic cancer. "Our 98% survival rate is among the highest in the country."[94]

3. Mayo Clinic (Rochester, MN)

"Mayo Clinic surgeons are experts in the Whipple procedure, every variation of it, and other pancreatic operations.

---

93. NYU Langone News. (2023). A leading surgeon helps patients with pancreatic cancer overcome steep odds. https://nyulangone.org/news/leading-surgeon-helps-patients-pancreatic-cancer-overcome-steep-odds
94. Duke Health. (2018, September 25). Whipple surgery for pancreatic cancer. https://www.dukehealth.org/blog/whipple-surgery-pancreatic-cancer

Each year Mayo Clinic surgeons perform over 450 such surgeries."[95]

Neoadjuvant and Adjuvant Treatment

Neoadjuvant treatment is therapy given before the main treatment, and it's often used for many kinds of cancers, including pancreatic cancer. The goal is to make the tumor smaller and fight cancer cells that might have spread but can't be seen yet. This can help doctors remove the whole tumor during surgery and could help the patient live longer.

Adjuvant chemotherapy is also given after surgery to destroy any leftover cancer cells. The aim is to lower the chances of the cancer coming back. One study found that in patients after surgery treated with "mFOLFIRINOX, a chemotherapy regimen containing four different medicines, lived a median of 20 months longer and were cancer-free nine months longer than those who received the current standard of care, gemcitabine (Gemzar®)."[96]

Here are some types of neoadjuvant and adjuvant treatments for pancreatic cancer. These treatments can be used by themselves or mixed together:

---

95. Mayo Foundation for Medical Education and Research. (2022, November 30). Whipple procedure. *Mayo Clinic.* https://www.mayoclinic.org/tests-procedures/whipple-procedure/care-at-mayo-clinic/pcc-20385056
96. ASCO. (2018, June 4). Chemotherapy regimen extends life by nearly twenty months for people with pancreatic cancer. https://old-prod.asco.org/about-asco/press-center/news-releases/chemotherapy-regimen-extends-life-nearly-twenty-months-people

- **Chemotherapy:** This uses special drugs to destroy cancer cells. Different combinations of drugs can be used depending on the patient's health and the type of tumor.

- **Radiation Therapy:** This uses powerful rays to kill cancer cells. Sometimes, it's used with chemotherapy. Dr. Amol Narang at Johns Hopkins says, "Combining chemotherapy and stereotactic radiation therapy in patients with pancreatic cancers that have attached to blood vessels shrinks the tumor, pulling it away from these critical vessels and making surgery possible for more patients."[97]

- **Targeted Therapies and Immunotherapies:** These treatments work in more specific ways. They either go after specific parts of cancer cells or help boost the body's own defenses against cancer.

After the neoadjuvant treatment, doctors will check the tumor again with scans and/or a biopsy to see if the therapy worked. If the tumor is a lot smaller and the patient is healthy enough, then the doctors can perform surgery to remove what's left of the tumor.

Choosing to use neoadjuvant therapy is a big decision. The surgeon leads this decision, but they should work closely with a team of doctors and the patient. Together, they need to consider the seriousness of the cancer, the patient's overall health, and

---

97. Johns Hopkins Medicine. (2018, December 26). Radiation therapy: Making inoperable cancers operable. https://www.hopkinsmedicine.org/news/articles/radiation-therapy

the patient's preferences. This way, they can figure out the best treatment and surgery plan as a team.[98]

Should you save some of your cancer cells from surgery by freezing them or later growing them into an organoid to study?

The reason you're having surgery really matters in answer to this question. If the surgery is for palliative care, which aims to ease symptoms but not cure the cancer, discussing the possibility of studying an organoid with your doctor can be important. In these cases, studying an organoid might provide valuable insights that could potentially improve your treatment outcomes. Therefore, considering the creation of an organoid could be beneficial in such situations.

If you have surgery to remove the whole tumor in pancreatic cancer, usually the cells are not used to make organoids or frozen for later, but they can be given to scientists for research. It's important to know that if your cancer comes back, the new cancer will probably be significantly different from the first one. So, if you've had successful surgery and then your cancer returns, your doctors will need to come up with a new treatment plan.

---

98. OpenAI. (2023). ChatGPT [Computer software]. Retrieved from https://www.openai.com/

Step Nine: Consider a Biopsy for an Organoid Before Starting Treatment

If the first round of chemotherapy is not effective... [Dr.] Demyan says, "you've already lost that critical window of opportunity to treat cancer... it's spreading very quickly."... CSHL [Cold Spring Harbor Laboratories] researchers found organoids can help guide pancreatic cancer patients' initial chemotherapy. CSHL runs one of the largest cancer organoid facilities in the country.[99]

Organoids act a lot like the real cancer in your body. This means scientists can test different drugs on it to see which ones work best, helping doctors choose the best first chemo for you. It's best if your cancer doctor picks your first chemo treatment based on information that's specific to you. As of summer 2023, this is still experimental.

---

99. Michalowski, J. (2022a, November 15). How organoids can guide pancreatic cancer therapy. Cold Spring Harbor Laboratory. https://www.cshl.edu/how-organoids-can-guide-pancreatic-cancer-therapy/

Progress has already been made at Cold Spring Harbor Laboratories (CSHL). It used to take several weeks to grow an organoid.

They piloted a rapid organoid screening test that can yield results in as early as a week. Getting quick results is important because pancreatic cancer patients usually do best if they undergo chemotherapy to shrink their tumor prior to surgery.[100]

CSHL shared their research on 117 people in a respected science journal. They successfully created organoids for about 75% of these patients in just one week. In their own words, the study "... correlated with PDO [Patient Derived Organoids] chemotherapy response..."[101] This means the organoids predicted how well the patients reacted to their first cancer medicine. Don't forget to talk about this choice with your cancer doctor.

In the "Hope" chapter, we talked about organoids. Again, think of them as a live mini-version of your cancer that scientists grow using your own cells in their lab. Even though they

---

100. Michalowski, J. (2022a, November 15). How organoids can guide pancreatic cancer therapy. Cold Spring Harbor Laboratory. https://www.cshl.edu/how-organoids-can-guide-pancreatic-cancer-therapy/
101. Demyan, L., Habowski, A. N., Plenker, D., King, D. A., Standring, O. J., Tsang, C., St Surin, L., Rishi, A., Crawford, J. M., Boyd, J., Pasha, S. A., Patel, H., Galluzzo, Z., Metz, C., Gregersen, P. K., Fox, S., Valente, C., Abadali, S., Matadial-Ragoo, S., DePeralta, D. K., Deutsch, G. B., Herman, J. M., Talamini, M. A., Tuveson, D. A., Weiss, M. J. (2022). Pancreatic cancer patient-derived organoids can predict response to neoadjuvant chemotherapy. *Annals of Surgery, 276*(3), 450-462. https://doi.org/10.1097/SLA.0000000000005558

don't look like a pancreas, organoids help scientists find out which medicines will work best for you.

It's best to do this before you start any chemo. But even if you've already started treatment, making an organoid is still possible. A study found that if you have chemo before taking cells to grow an organoid, it only makes it 5% less likely to work.[102]

If you found out you have pancreatic cancer through a biopsy but didn't know about organoids back then, it's okay. You can ask for another biopsy. For those whose cancer has moved to their liver, getting a biopsy from the liver is easier than from the pancreas. These liver cells are actually just pancreatic cancer cells that have traveled, so they're basically the same. The more live cells that get collected, the faster scientists can make and test the organoid. Getting a liver biopsy is a good idea because it's easier and helps with collecting more cells, which makes the whole process quicker.

You can even grow an organoid from simple blood test, called a liquid biopsy. But there are some challenges. The test collects only a few cancer cells. Growing these cells into bigger samples for study takes time. Despite these issues, the liquid biopsy can still provide valuable information for treating cancer.

---

102. Demyan, L., Habowski, A. N., Plenker, D., King, D. A., Standring, O. J., Tsang, C., St Surin, L., Rishi, A., Crawford, J. M., Boyd, J., Pasha, S. A., Patel, H., Galluzzo, Z., Metz, C., Gregersen, P. K., Fox, S., Valente, C., Abadali, S., Matadial-Ragoo, S., DePeralta, D. K., Deutsch, G. B., Herman, J. M., Talamini, M. A., Tuveson, D. A., Weiss, M. J. (2022). Pancreatic cancer patient-derived organoids can predict response to neoadjuvant chemotherapy. *Annals of Surgery, 276*(3), 450-462. https://doi.org/10.1097/SLA.0000000000005558

Organoids can be really pricey ($$$) if you can even find a commercial lab to grow and test them. Your health insurance will probably not pay for it. To make it less expensive, you can look for special studies called clinical trials that use organoids. These could be more affordable. One example is the PASS-01 trial led by Dr. David Tuveson at Cold Spring Harbor Laboratory. This study uses organoids to help people with pancreatic cancer.[103]

Antabuse is a drug that helps slow down the growth of pancreatic cancer in some people. This was found out through organoid research. It's been used for many years to help people stop drinking alcohol. Some early experiments with organoids showed that Antabuse can either kill or drastically slow down the growth of pancreatic cancer in a lot of people.[104] Plus, if you take Antabuse with a copper supplement, it can make radiation therapy work better.[105]

The good news is that since Antabuse is already approved and available by prescription in pharmacies there, doctors can prescribe it. But there's one important warning: if you're taking Antabuse, you can't drink any alcohol at all, not even a tiny sip. If you do, you could feel very sick and start throwing up.

---

103. Michalowski, J. (2022a, November 15). How organoids can guide pancreatic cancer therapy. Cold Spring Harbor Laboratory. https://www.cshl.edu/how-organoids-can-guide-pancreatic-cancer-therapy/

104. Dastjerdi, M. N., Babazadeh, Z., Rabbani, M., Gharagozloo, M., Esmaeili, A., & Narimani, M. (2014). Effects of disulfiram on apoptosis in PANC-1 human pancreatic cancer cell line. *Research in Pharmaceutical Sciences, 9*(4), 287-294.

105. Xu, Y., Lu, L., Luo, J., Wang, L., Zhang, Q., Cao, J., & Jiao, Y. (2021). Disulfiram alone functions as a radiosensitizer for pancreatic cancer both in vitro and in vivo. *Frontiers in Oncology, 11*, Article 683695. https://doi.org/10.3389/fonc.2021.683695

Organoids are helpful, but they're not perfect or ready for everyone to use yet. As I write this book in summer 2023, you have to sign up for a clinical trial to use organoids. But things might change in the future. By the time you read this, there may be companies that make it easy to get organoids made from your own cancer cells.

This important work was started by Dr. David Tuveson from Cold Spring Harbor Laboratory and Dr. Hans Clevers from the Dutch Science Foundation. The Lustgarten Foundation is helping to pay for this research on organoids made from pancreatic tumors. Also, the Herbert Wertheim UF Scripps Institute for Biomedical Innovation & Technology has been a leader in research about how to test the organoids, called high-throughput testing.

To find out where studies are happening, you'll need to search online for the term "pancreatic cancer organoid clinical research." Many schools and research labs are focused on studying organoids for pancreatic cancer. Here are some of the big names working on it:

- **Cold Spring Harbor Laboratory**—The Tuveson lab at Cold Spring Harbor Laboratory is seriously into studying pancreatic cancer using organoids. They look at how these mini-organs work and how different the cancer cells can be, and they're also trying to come up with new treatments for pancreatic cancer.

  Websites: https://www.cshl.edu/ and https://tuvesonlab.labsites.cshl.edu/

- **The Organoid Group at the Hubrecht Institute**—The Netherlands is a leader in organoid research. They've made pancreatic organoids and are using them to study how pancreatic cancer gets worse over time, why some treatments stop working, and how to find the best medicines to fight the cancer.

    Websites: https://www.hubrecht.eu/ and https://www.hubrecht.eu/research-groups/clevers-group/

- **Harvard University**—The Muthuswamy laboratory was among the first to employ three-dimensional cell culture (now referred to as organoid culture) to bridge the gap between growing cells as a flat monolayer and tumors growing *in vivo*. They apply a microscope-to-stethoscope approach that combines basic cell biology investigations with clinical translation, as evidenced by the successful completion of a clinical trial: Harnessing Organoids for Personalized therapy (HOPE) in pancreatic cancer.[106]

    Website: https://ccr.cancer.gov/staff-directory/senthil-k-muthuswamy/lab

- **MIT (Massachusetts Institute of Technology) and Cancer Research UK Manchester Institute**—MIT engineers, in collaboration with scientists at Cancer Research UK Manchester Institute, have developed a new way to grow tiny replicas of the pancreas, using either healthy

---

106. Muthuswamy Lab. (2023). Muthuswamy Lab | Center for Cancer Research. Retrieved from https://ccr.cancer.gov/staff-directory/senthil-k-muthuswamy/lab

or cancerous pancreatic cells. Their new models could help researchers develop and test potential drugs for pancreatic cancer, which is currently one of the most difficult types of cancer to treat.[107]

Websites: https://ki.mit.edu/ and https://www.cruk.manchester.ac.uk/

- **Johns Hopkins University**—Scientists at Johns Hopkins University are using organoids to learn more about pancreatic cancer. They are trying to find out how to detect this cancer early on, understand the different types of cells in the tumors, and create more personalized treatments.

    Website: https://www.hopkinsmedicine.org/surgery/specialty-areas/hepato-pancreato-biliary-hpb-surgery/research/organoid-research

- **University of California, San Francisco (UCSF)**—The research team led by Prof. Matthias Hebrok at the University of California, San Francisco (UCSF) is also studying organoids. They want to learn how pancreatic cancer starts, gets worse over time, and spreads to other parts of the body.

    Website: https://rooselab.ucsf.edu/organoids.html

---

107. Trafton, A. (2021, September 13). Engineers grow pancreatic "organoids" that mimic the real thing. MIT News | Massachusetts Institute of Technology. https://news.mit.edu/2021/pancreatic-organoids-cancer-0913

- **Keio University School of Medicine**—Research about pancreatic organoids has been led by Dr. Toshiro Sato.[108]

  Email: t.sato@keio.jp

- **Sumitomo Pharma**[109]

  Website: https://www.sumitomo-pharma.com/

- **The First Hospital of Lanzhou University, The First Clinical Medical School of Lanzhou University**— Research about pancreatic organoids has been led by Drs. Jia Yao and Man Yang[110]

This list of labs, schools and company above might not include all the places, especially in other countries, that are using organoids to learn about pancreatic cancer when this was written. There might be others. The field is changing and advancing quickly. Researchers are focused on understanding more about pancreatic cancer so they can come up with better treatments for it.

---

108. Seino, T., Kawasaki, S., Shimokawa, M., Tamagawa, H., Toshimitsu, K., Fujii, M., Ohta, Y., Matano, M., Nanki, K., Kawasaki, K., Takahashi, S., Sugimoto, S., Iwasaki, E., Takagi, J., Itoi, T., Kitago, M., Kitagawa, Y., Kanai, T., & Sato, T. (2018). Human pancreatic tumor organoids reveal loss of stem cell niche factor dependence during disease progression. *Cell Stem Cell, 22*(3), 454-457. https://doi.org/10.1016/j.stem.2017.12.009

109. Watanabe, S., Yogo, A., Otsubo, T., Umehara, H., Oishi, J., Kodo, T., Masui, T., Takaishi, S., Seno, H., Uemoto, S., & Hatano, E. (2022). Establishment of patient-derived organoids and a characterization-based drug discovery platform for treatment of pancreatic cancer. *BMC Cancer, 22*(1), Article 489. https://doi.org/10.1186/s12885-022-09619-9

110. Yao, J., Yang, M., Atteh, L., Liu, P., Mao, Y., Meng, W., & Li, X. (2021). A pancreas tumor derived organoid study: from drug screen to precision medicine. *Cancer Cell International, 21*(1), Article 398. https://doi.org/10.1186/s12935-021-02044-1

Step Ten: If Surgery Was Not an Option or Your Cancer Came Back After Surgery, Choose Your Treatment

No matter what job you do, someone who hasn't done that work can't become an expert just by searching on the internet for a few hours. Let's say, for example, say that someone wants to buy a new house. They find a house they like online that's in a good school district and is 25% cheaper than other similar houses. The house seems perfect when they visit it. But a real estate agent who really knows the local houses says that the wind isn't blowing from the north that day. If it were, you'd quickly notice a foul smell from a nearby trash dump. That's why the house is cheaper than others in the same school district.

Reading this book and other resources can help you learn more about pancreatic cancer and health care. But remember, just reading doesn't make you an expert overnight. When deciding on your first treatment, you need to trust your cancer doctor's advice. If you have doubts, get a second opinion. However, do not ignore the experts as Steve Jobs did.

According to AI, "The effectiveness of chemotherapy in extending the life of individuals with pancreatic cancer can vary significantly. This depends on several factors, including:

- the stage of the cancer,

- the patient's overall health,

- how the cancer responds to treatment."[111]

Chemotherapy is the main way to treat pancreatic cancer. It can help people live longer, maybe by a few months[112] or even up to two years.[113] However, how well it works depends on the factors listed above. Sadly, doctors don't expect it to cure advanced pancreatic cancer.[114] Another downside of chemotherapy is that it can make some people feel really sick. The hope

---

111. OpenAI. (2023). ChatGPT [Computer software]. Retrieved from https://www.openai.com/
112. Wainberg, Z. (2023, January 20). A 4-drug chemotherapy regimen improves survival in stage 4 pancreas cancer. UCLA Health. https://www.uclahealth.org/news/4-drug-chemotherapy-regimen-improves-survival-stage-4
113. Shaikh, J. (2023). Can pancreatic cancer be cured with chemotherapy? Moffitt Cancer Center. Retrieved from https://www.moffitt.org/cancers/pancreatic-cancer/faqs/can-pancreatic-cancer-be-cured-with-chemo/
114. Shaikh, J. (2023). Can pancreatic cancer be cured with chemotherapy? Moffitt Cancer Center. Retrieved from https://www.moffitt.org/cancers/pancreatic-cancer/faqs/can-pancreatic-cancer-be-cured-with-chemo/

is that chemotherapy can help people live long enough to try newer, better treatments later on.

I suggest "chemotherapy plus," a term and concept I learned from Dr. Allyson Ocean. It means traditional care plus additional treatments or supplements. What to choose for the "plus" is a decision you should make with the help of a well-qualified and open-minded oncologist and the team you have supporting you. Together, you should review all treatment options. As you choose what to add to your standard of care, use these guiding principles:

- **Make sure that you are doing no harm.** Some people take a large amount of vitamin C through an IV (like fifty grams) when they have chemotherapy, hoping it will make the side effects less severe. But there's a real worry that this vitamin C might actually weaken the chemotherapy's power to fight cancer, not just reduce its side effects.

- **Make no unforced errors.** I use this tennis term to say that you should avoid simple mistakes like not understanding the directions for taking a medicine or unintentionally missing a medical appointment. Double-check everything that you can. Use reminders for medications and upcoming appointments. Allow your team members to help you wherever possible. There is a lot that is out of your control about this disease. Concentrate on what you can get right and improve.

- **Have some scientific evidence, even if it's not conclusive.** This will be important to help you decide on treatments. Again, scientific evidence is found in medical journals and at medical conferences. Internet searches, AI searches, and websites can also help you find reliable information.

- **Use common sense.** This is a simple phrase that most people intuitively understand. Despite the fear and other emotions that you are likely feeling, you need to take a moment to reflect and use your best judgment before making any major decisions.

Jennifer Kennedy writes, "Pancreatic cancer is difficult to treat. There are a few standard treatments, but there are additional options that we encourage patients to consider."[115] Treating pancreatic cancer is like trying to balance on a tightrope. Chemotherapy is a powerful medicine that can be used on its own or with other treatments. Some chemo comes as a pill, and most types must be given through an IV, a tube that goes into a vein in your arm. While it can make people live longer, it can also make them feel really tired, sick to their stomach, lose their hair, and catch illnesses more easily. In rare cases, it might even harm important parts of the body like the heart or lungs.

There are also different treatments like targeted therapies, immunotherapies, or radiotherapy that are more focused. These treatments aim to attack just the cancer cells and leave the healthy cells alone. Usually, people feel better with these treatments compared to chemotherapy. But the downside is

---

115. Kennedy, J. (2017, October 18). Treatment options for pancreatic cancer patients beyond standard care. *Pancreatic Cancer Action Network*. https://pancan.org/news/going-beyond-standard-care/

that these treatments might not help people live as long as they would with chemotherapy.

Deciding on the right treatment is like choosing the best tool for a job. Doctors and patients need to talk about how far the cancer has spread, how healthy the patient is, and what the patient is comfortable with.

In simple terms, the decision is sometimes about choosing between living longer with more side effects or living for a shorter time with fewer side effects. It's a tough choice that needs to be made carefully.[116]

Just like a shoe store salesperson will try to sell you new shoes, medical experts might lean toward the treatments they know best and do in their practice. Each type of doctor is an expert in their own area, so they might suggest treatments that they're most familiar with.

That's another reason why it's important to talk to different kinds of specialists and get second opinion(s). This will help you see the full picture of all the treatment options. It can also be helpful to do your own research and ask lots of questions so you can make the best decision for you. Remember, it's your health, so you have the final say in how you want to be treated.

---

116. OpenAI. (2023). ChatGPT [Computer software]. Retrieved from https://www.openai.com/

Consider Chemotherapy

Chemotherapy drugs can be seen as poisons that specifically target cells that divide rapidly. These drugs travel throughout your entire body, which has its pros and cons. On the positive side, they can treat very small metastases that are too tiny to be detected.[117]

Cancer cells multiply super-fast, but they aren't the only ones in our bodies doing this. Most of the cells in an adult's body aren't multiplying (getting bigger and then splitting) much. But some important cells are different. Cells inside our bones constantly make new blood cells—white and red. The cells that make our hair grow are quick to multiply, too. Cells in our digestive system, which begin in our mouth and extend to our large intestine, constantly create new cells. This process helps our body to function well and allows us to absorb nutrients from the food we eat. These cells naturally fall off when food and waste move through our system. The problem is chemotherapy drugs can't tell these fast-dividing cells from cancer cells. As a result, these drugs sometimes harm these healthy cells as well.

Oncologists have a responsibility to ensure your chemotherapy treatment matches the "standard of care." This standard is set by cancer specialists in the state where they practice, because doctors receive their licenses from the state government. Although cancer treatment might vary slightly from one state to another, it's generally quite similar across the board.

---

117. Texas Oncology. (2017). Stage IV pancreatic cancer. Retrieved May 30, 2017, from https://www.texasoncology.com/types-of-cancer/pancreatic-cancer/stage-iv-pancreatic-cancer/. Reprinted with permission.

Put simply, the standard of care reflects what most doctors would do if they were faced with a similar situation. This standard often comes from the findings of clinical trials, which are typically conducted with great care and precision.[118]

Understanding Clinical Trials and AI in Pancreatic Cancer Treatment

Clinical trials, like randomized controlled trials (RCTs), play a crucial role in discovering effective treatments for pancreatic cancer. They're considered the best method for testing new treatments. However, these trials face several challenges:

- **Cost:** Clinical trials are expensive due to the extensive resources required, such as staffing, equipment, and patient care. According to the NIH, the median cost in 2015-2017 was $48 million.[119] The Association of Community Cancer Centers says that the total cost for an oncology study in the U.S. was about $79 million in 2015.[120] "In 2015, the Pharmaceutical Research and Manufacturers of America

---

118. Goguen, D. (n.d.). What is the medical standard of care? Medical malpractice lawsuits stem from a medical professional's deviation from this legal obligation that they owe their patients. http://www.alllaw.com/articles/nolo/medical-malpractice/standard-of-care.html
119. Moore, T. J., Heyward, J., Anderson, G., & Alexander, G. C. (2020). Variation in the estimated costs of pivotal clinical benefit trials supporting the US approval of new therapeutic agents, 2015-2017: a cross-sectional study. *BMJ open, 10*(6), e038863. https://doi.org/10.1136/bmjopen-2020-038863
120. Association of Community Cancer Centers. (n.d.). Clinical trials in immunotherapy. Retrieved from https://www.accc-cancer.org

(PhRMA) published... oncology trials showed the highest average per-patient cost, with an average per-patient cost of $59,500."[121,122]

- **Time:** The journey from the start of a clinical trial to the adoption of its findings into standard care is long. This process involves several stages, including planning, approval, patient enrollment, and data analysis. "There is no typical length of time it takes for a drug to be tested and approved. It might take 10 to 15 years or more to complete all 3 phases of clinical trials before the licensing stage. But this time span varies a lot."[123] An initiative like the PanCAN's Precision Promise^{SM} aims to speed up this process by using adaptive clinical trial designs, which allow for more efficient testing of new therapies.[124]

- **Lack of Inclusivity:** Traditional clinical trials often struggle with inclusivity, typically enrolling a limited demographic that doesn't fully represent the broader patient population. Although specific statistics on participation demographics

---

121. Association of Community Cancer Centers. (n.d.). Clinical trials in immunotherapy. Retrieved from https://www.accc-cancer.org
122. ACM Global Laboratories. (2024). How to plan for a successful oncology clinical trial. https://www.acmgloballab.com/about-us/resources/oncology-clinical-trial
123. Cancer Research UK. (2022, February 1). How long a new drug takes to go through clinical trials. https://www.cancerresearchuk.org/about-cancer/find-a-clinical-trial/how-clinical-trials-are-planned-and-organised/how-long-it-takes-for-a-new-drug-to-go-through-clinical-trials
124. Pancreatic Cancer Action Network. (2024, January 10). Pancan's precision promise adaptive clinical trial platform. Retrieved from https://pancan.org/research/precision-promise/

were not found, it's acknowledged that enhancing diversity in clinical trials is a critical goal for improving research outcomes and equity. "Only 3-5% of cancer patients in the United States participate in a cancer CT [Clinical Trials] and there are disparities in CT participation by age, race and gender."[125] In their study on the enrollment of racial minorities in clinical trials, Nazha et al. (2019) in "Enrollment of Racial Minorities in Clinical Trials: Old Problem Assumes New Urgency in the Age of Immunotherapy," highlight the significant underrepresentation of these groups:

> An analysis of 1 million patients with cancer in the United States showed that blacks or African Americans have a 28% higher cancer-specific mortality compared with whites. This survival gap is independent of sociodemographic factors, disease stage, and access to treatments... It is well established that U.S. patients of minority racial/ethnic backgrounds have a level of willingness to participate in clinical trials that is comparable to that of whites... Contemporary oncology trials continue to be characterized by an overrepresentation of white and male. participants (80% and 59.8%, respectively).[126]

Lee and Wen (2020), in their study "Gender and Sex Disparity in Cancer Trials" published in ESMO Open, address the

---

125. Cartmell, K. B., Bonilha, H. S., Simpson, K. N., Ford, M. E., Bryant, D. C., & Alberg, A. J. (2020). Patient barriers to cancer clinical trial participation and navigator activities to assist. *Advances in cancer research, 146*, 139-166. https://doi.org/10.1016/bs.acr.2020.01.008

126. Bassel Nazha et al., Enrollment of Racial Minorities in Clinical Trials: Old Problem Assumes New Urgency in the Age of Immunotherapy. *Am Soc Clin Oncol Educ Book 39, 3-10*(2019). doi:10.1200/EDBK_100021

significant disparities in cancer trial participation among different genders and sexes:

> ... women are still under-represented in cancer trials. Of the 5157 patients who participated in oncology trials that led to the FDA approval of 17 new drugs in 2018, only 38% were women... females were under-represented in lung cancer, melanoma and pancreatic cancer trials despite the higher prevalence of these cancers in females.[127]

AI in healthcare offers promising alternatives to traditional research methods by addressing some of these challenges:

- **Cost-Effectiveness:** AI can analyze large datasets from electronic medical records at a lower cost compared to traditional clinical trials, although specific cost comparisons were not obtained. This efficiency could enable more extensive and inclusive research within limited budgets. Exact cost data is impossible to find but AI says:

    > As a rough estimate, off-the-shelf AI solutions for healthcare data analysis can start at a few thousand dollars per year in subscription fees for small-scale implementations. Custom solutions can range from tens of thousands to hundreds of thousands of dollars, depending on the project's complexity and scale.

---

127. Lee, E., & Wen, P. (2020). Gender and sex disparity in cancer trials. *ESMO open, 5*(Suppl 4), e000773. https://doi.org/10.1136/esmoopen-2020-000773

- **Speed:** AI technologies can process and analyze data much faster than human researchers, potentially accelerating the pace at which new discoveries are made and applied to patient care. Again, exact information is hard to find but AI estimates, "Overall, for a moderately complex project, you might expect a timeline from about 3 to 6 months from start to finish."

- **Inclusivity:** By easily using lots of data including that from diverse populations in electronic medical records, AI research can include a broader range of demographic groups, enhancing the relevance and applicability of its findings across different patient backgrounds.

- **Capability:** AI's ability to analyze complex genetic information, including the role of thousands of genes in cancer, offers a deeper understanding of disease mechanisms that could lead to more personalized and effective treatments. Although specific examples of AI analyzing all 22,000 active genes in cancer were not found, the potential for AI to manage such complex data is a significant advantage over traditional research methods. Such an approach would not only facilitate the analysis of existing data but also set the stage for expanded testing opportunities such as the from testing pancreatic cancer organoids.

AI's application in healthcare is expanding, from analyzing lab test results to identifying new therapeutic targets in organoids, demonstrating its potential to transform cancer research and treatment by making it more efficient, inclusive, and cost-effective. Basically, what AI does is search for patterns and connections between data and positive results.

Are we trying to compare two very different things, like apples and oranges? In a way, yes, and in another way, no. Randomized controlled trials continue to be the only safe and recognized method for discovering new drugs. However, artificial intelligence is also uncovering new and improved methods for treating conditions like pancreatic diseases. While AI research offers numerous benefits, as of early 2024, it sometimes produces inaccurate or misleading information. As a result, it's crucial that doctors and scientists thoroughly review AI findings. AI represents a groundbreaking and necessary tool. It's not a replacement for medical professionals or traditional scientific methods but rather a vital resource to address the immediate needs of people with pancreatic cancer.

Sometimes, such as with information from AI, there can be more than one way to solve a health problem that fits within the accepted rules of medicine. Doctors might worry about getting sued if they make a mistake. But the law gives doctors some wiggle-room to use their judgment when making decisions. This is known as the "second school of thought" or "respected minority opinion." It means that even if most doctors would pick one way of doing things, choosing a different way could still be okay if there's a good reason.

Your treatment for any health problem should be personalized, considering your unique situation and your own preferences. It's important, though, that your doctor's plan is carefully thought out and based on good information.[128] So, your oncologist has some flexibility but only within guidelines.

As of summer 2023, chemotherapy is used to treat most pancreatic cancer cases that have spread to other parts of the body. It's important to remember that just because chemotherapy is the standard or usual treatment, it doesn't mean it's always the best for everyone. New ways to treat this cancer are always being explored.

Treatments, like drugs or other methods, have to be approved by the US Food and Drug Administration (FDA) before they can be used. To become the new standard of care, a therapy has to be shown to work better than the current standard treatment. This is a tough requirement to meet, but it helps ensure that new treatments really are improvements over the old ones.

In summary, from AI, chemotherapy:

Pros:

- Fighting the Cancer: Chemo can shrink the tumor, slow the cancer's growth, and kill any cancer cells that may have spread to other parts of the body. This can make a person feel better and live longer.

---

128. Goguen, D. (n.d.). What is the medical standard of care? Medical malpractice lawsuits stem from a medical professional's deviation from this legal obligation that they owe their patients. http://www.alllaw.com/articles/nolo/medical-malpractice/standard-of-care.html

- Before or After Surgery: Sometimes, doctors use chemo before surgery to make a big tumor smaller, which makes it easier to remove. It can also be used after surgery to kill any leftover cancer cells.

Cons:

- Side Effects: The big downside of chemo is that it can have some tough side effects. These can include feeling very tired, losing hair, feeling nauseated (like you're going to throw up), or having a low appetite. This happens because chemo drugs can't tell the difference between cancer cells and healthy cells, so they also end up hurting some healthy cells.

- Not Always Effective: Unfortunately, chemo doesn't always work. Pancreatic cancer is known for being tough to treat, and sometimes the cancer cells don't respond to the drugs.[129]

Consider Radiation Oncologist's Opinion

Radiation therapy (RT) isn't usually the first choice for treating pancreatic cancer that has spread to other parts of the body (metastatic pancreatic cancer). But it can be used alone or together with other treatments like chemotherapy.

---

129. OpenAI. (2023). ChatGPT [Computer software]. Retrieved from https://www.openai.com/

RT works in a unique way, like a sniper targeting cancer. It wipes out cancer cells in the area it's aimed at. But RT has challenges just as surgery has. The pancreas is located deep inside our body, close to important organs like the stomach, intestines, and big blood vessels. RT could accidentally harm these parts of the body, just as a surgeon's knife can cut the wrong thing.

The pancreas's location makes it tough to use radiation treatments without risking harm to healthy body parts nearby. Here's how RT works: It shoots beams of radiation from different directions at the cancer cells. Each beam is carefully controlled to keep the healthy tissue safe. But where these beams cross, they create a high-powered dose of radiation that destroys the cancer cells.

RT can also be used to shrink larger cancers. This can prevent them from blocking the pancreas or bile ducts, which are tubes that help with digestion.

RT is a way to treat cancer without using strong drugs like those in chemotherapy. People like it because the side effects are often not as bad. You might feel tired, not want to eat, or even feel a little sick, but it's generally easier to handle than chemotherapy.

In radiation therapy, doctors use special machines to send X-rays or other energy beams right at the tumor. This helps to kill off the cancer cells. There are different types of radiation therapy, so you have options on how to get treated:

1. **Conventional external-beam RT:** It is a type of radiation therapy in which you go to the hospital or clinic usu-

ally five days per week for about five weeks to get your treatment. They use a machine to aim X-rays right at your tumor. You get a little bit of treatment each day instead of a lot all at once. This helps the healthy parts around the tumor to heal between your visits. That way, there's less chance of hurting the healthy parts of your body and you're less likely to have bad side effects.

2. **High-dose RT (stereotactic):** Sometimes called "radiosurgery," "cybersurgery," or "gamma knife," is a stronger kind of radiation therapy. Instead of going for many days, you only go for four to six sessions. Because it's stronger, there's a higher chance you might have more serious side effects. But this method can be a good choice for older people who can't have surgery and whose pancreatic cancer has come back in just one area. Dr. Wei and his colleagues write, "Gamma knife stereotactic radiosurgery has the advantage in protecting the surrounding tissues and providing short-term effects."[130]

3. **Intensity-modulated and image-guided RT:** These are fancy types of radiation therapy that use special technology to be highly accurate. These types are usually only found at certain places like big hospitals or special cancer centers. The machines make sure the X-rays go exactly where they're needed, which helps to protect the healthy parts of your body.

---

130. Wei, J., Dong, X., Du, F., Tang, S., & Wei, H. (2017). Successful gamma knife radiosurgery combined with S-1 in an elderly man with local recurrent pancreatic cancer: A case report. *Medicine (Baltimore), 96*(51), e9338. https://doi.org/10.1097/MD.0000000000009338

Whether or not this is the best option for you depends on your specific situation with pancreatic cancer. Your doctors can help you decide if it's a good fit.

4. **Brachytherapy:** is another way to treat tumors using radiation, but it's a bit different because the radiation source is placed close to the tumor or even inside it. There are two main kinds:

   A. **Temporary brachytherapy:** In temporary brachytherapy, a special device is put close to or inside the cancer to give radiation. This device is taken out after the treatment and isn't left inside the body. The time the radiation is given can be different. If it's a high dose, the radiation might only take about 10 to 20 minutes, but it can be given more than once over a few weeks.

   If it's a low dose, the radiation goes on for a longer time, like 20 to 50 hours, and you might have to stay in the hospital while it's happening. Both high dose rate (HDR) and low dose rate (LDR) brachytherapy techniques can be used in the treatment of pancreatic cancer.

   B. **Permanent brachytherapy:** Tiny metal seeds are put right into the tumor. These seeds give off a weaker dose of radiation but stay there for a long time, like several days. This is often used for big tumors that have spread to the liver. There's a special example called the Y-90 procedure, which you can learn about in the next section.

Both methods try to focus the radiation right where it's needed, which helps to leave the healthy parts of your body alone.

If you're thinking about getting radiation therapy, you can talk to your regular doctor or your oncologist to find a radiation therapy doctor who can help you. Another way to find a good radiation therapy doctor is by checking the *U.S. News & World Report* website. They have rankings and information that can help you make a choice.[131]

The coverage of appointments with radiation therapy specialists for pancreatic cancer treatment can vary depending on the patient's insurance plan. Radiation oncologists, who specialize in treating cancer with radiation therapy, play a crucial role in the multidisciplinary approach to pancreatic cancer treatment. However, they are not typically the first specialists that patients see for their treatment, which may affect insurance coverage for their consultations.

You should see a radiation oncologist before starting chemotherapy for the following reasons:

- Your cancer might be unique in a way that makes treatment with radiation, instead of drugs, a better option.

- There might have been advancements or upgrades in how RT is done since this book was written.

---

131. U.S. News & World Report. (2023). Find radiation oncologists | US News Doctors—US News Health. Find Radiation Oncologists. Retrieved from https://health.usnews.com/doctors/location-index/radiation-oncologists

- Radiation oncologists often have different ideas about treating pancreatic cancer than medical oncologists, who use medicines like chemotherapy. Even if radiation therapy isn't right for you, a radiation oncologist might have other suggestions that could still help in your treatment. So, it's a good idea to get their opinion.

Consider an Interventional Radiology Opinion

Before you decide on a treatment plan, consider having a chat with a doctor known as an interventional radiologist. They might suggest a treatment called the Y-90 procedure. This method is a special type of x-ray/radiation treatment that uses something called intra-arterial yttrium-90 radioembolization.

What happens during this treatment? The doctor will put tiny radioactive beads (only about five times bigger than a red blood cell) into any liver growths from pancreatic cancer. These beads are not harmful and help fight the cancer cells in your liver.

After a Y-90 procedure, patients might still feel some symptoms. However, for patients whose pancreatic cancer has spread to the liver, a Y-90 treatment can really help. It can lessen cancer symptoms in your liver and even help you live longer. This is important because when someone dies from pancreatic cancer, it's most often because of liver failure.

Radioembolization is a treatment that can't cure pancreatic

cancer but can help people feel better and live longer.[132] Compared to a tough treatment like chemotherapy, it's generally easier on the body. For example, you might feel extremely tired after some chemotherapy treatments for a week to ten days. But with radioembolization, you usually won't feel as tired, and other side effects are often not as severe.[133]

Consider Immune System Based Treatments

Immunotherapy is a special kind of treatment that uses your body's own defenses. It boosts your body's defense system to help it fight cancer. Your doctor can either give you vaccines, drugs, and supplements to improve your immune system function. Or they can take some of your immune cells out with a blood draw, strengthen them in the lab, and give them back to you. Immunotherapy helps in several ways:

- It can slow down or stop cancer cells from growing.

- It can prevent cancer from spreading to different parts of your body.

- It can strengthen your immune system and help it kill cancer cells.

---

132. Y-90 liver cancer-busting treatment: Safe, fast, extends life, study finds. (2011, March 28). *Science Daily.* https://www.sciencedaily.com/releases/2011/03/110328092409.htm

133. Y-90 liver cancer-busting treatment: Safe, fast, extends life, study finds. (2011, March 28). *Science Daily.* https://www.sciencedaily.com/releases/2011/03/110328092409.htm

Ideally, immunotherapy has some big benefits. For example, it can travel all over your body and destroy tiny groups of cancer cells that may have spread, known as microscopic metastases. Researchers are always studying and learning more about it. Another good thing is that usually "it causes fewer side effects than other treatments."[134] As Stephanie Booth writes for WebMD, "these side effects are different for everyone. They depend on the specific type of immunotherapy you receive, the type of cancer you have, its location, your general health, and other factors."[135]

But there's a downside, too. Even though a lot of these immune-based treatments sound great in theory, they have not performed as well as doctors expected/hoped when tested in large studies. "Right now, immunotherapy works for fewer than half the people who try it. Many people only have a partial response."[136]

The immune system has two basic components. The T-cell is a type of white blood cell circulating in your blood. T-cells can be considered soldier cells because they can directly kill cancer cells. The second component is antibodies, which are proteins that circulate in the blood like cruise missiles. These proteins specifically target one thing that can harm the body. For

---

134. Booth, S. (2023, March 12). What are the pros and cons of immunotherapy? WebMD. https://www.webmd.com/cancer/immunotherapy-risks-benefits

135. Side effects of immunotherapy. (2022, May 1). Cancer.Net. https://www.cancer.net/navigating-cancer-care/how-cancer-treated/immunotherapy-and-vaccines/side-effects-immunotherapy

136. Booth, S. (2023, March 12). What are the pros and cons of immunotherapy? WebMD. https://www.webmd.com/cancer/immunotherapy-risks-benefits

instance, immunizations such as the flu shot cause the body to make antibodies to kill flu viruses if they infect you.

There are many types of immunotherapies. Here are a few:

- **Natural and Lab-Developed Antibodies (Researched Using AI)**[137]

    Scientists are studying two kinds of antibodies to fight pancreatic cancer. First, there are natural antibodies in our bodies. Researchers found that people with pancreatic cancer have lower levels of a specific natural antibodies against a natural chemical, 3'-sialyllactose, compared to healthy people. By measuring these antibody levels, doctors might be able to spot pancreatic cancer early.[138]

    Second, scientists in labs are making special antibodies to target pancreatic cancer. They've created a new kind, called a bispecific nanobody, which attacks specific parts of cancer cells. This is still being tested, but it's showing some promise in helping to treat pancreatic cancer.[139]

---

137. OpenAI. (2023). ChatGPT [Computer software]. Retrieved from https://www.openai.com/
138. Yamada, K., Higashi, K., Nagahori, H., & Saito, K. (2020). Circulating natural antibodies against 3'-sialyllactose complement the diagnostic performance of CA19-9 for the early detection of pancreatic ductal adenocarcinoma. *Cancer biomarkers : section A of Disease markers, 27*(1), 121-128. https://doi.org/10.3233/CBM-190158
139. Hao, S., Xu, S., Li, L. et al. Tumour inhibitory activity on pancreatic cancer by bispecific nanobody targeting PD-L1 and CXCR4. *BMC Cancer 22*, 1092 (2022). https://doi.org/10.1186/s12885-022-10165-7

However, it's important to know that many of these new antibody treatments are still being studied and haven't yet been proven to work really well. Researchers are hopeful and continue to look for better ways to use these antibodies against pancreatic cancer.[140]

- **Monoclonal antibody/checkpoint inhibitor**

In July 2020, the FDA said it's okay to use a medicine called Keytruda for more people with pancreatic cancer. If your cancer doctor tells you your tumor has a "high tumor mutational burden,"[141] you can get Keytruda as a treatment. Before this change, only 1% to 2% of patients could get it. They had to have one of two special things in their tumor—either mismatch repair deficiency or microsatellite instability.

The "... immune checkpoint inhibitor pembrolizumab [brand name Keytruda] is the only immunotherapy that is FDA-approved for the treatment of patients with advanced PDAC [pancreatic ductal adenocarcinoma]."[142]

---

140. Kaur, J., Singh, P., Enzler, T., & Sahai, V. (2021). Emerging antibody therapies for pancreatic adenocarcinoma: a review of recent phase 2 trials. *Expert opinion on emerging drugs, 26*(2), 103-129. https://doi.org/10.1080/14728214.2021.1905795
141. Sharpless, N. E. (2020, July 8). Pembrolizumab FDA approval and genomic testing in cancer. National Cancer Institute. https://www.cancer.gov/news-events/cancer-currents-blog/2020/fda-pembrolizumab-tmb-approval-genomic-testing
142. Bian, J., & Almhanna, K. (2021). Pancreatic cancer and immune checkpoint inhibitors—still a long way to go. *Translational Gastroenterology and Hepatology, 6*, Article 6. https://doi.org/10.21037/tgh.2020.04.03

- **Cancer vaccines**

    As of summer 2023, scientists are still studying vaccines for cancer. These vaccines aren't available for everyone yet; they're only in clinical trials. Unlike the vaccines we usually get to prevent diseases, a vaccine for pancreatic cancer wouldn't stop you from getting the cancer in the first place. Instead, it would be used to help treat people who already have this type of cancer.[143]

    A very hopeful study was done at Memorial Sloan Kettering and published in a science magazine called *Nature*. They teamed up with a company named BioNTech to make a special kind of vaccine using mRNA technology. This is the same technology used in the Pfizer and Moderna Covid vaccines. The exciting news is that in the test, 8 out of 19 patients did not have their cancer return for 18 months after surgery.[144]

---

143. Zheng, L. (Ed.). (2022, April 5). Pancreatic cancer vaccine: What to know. Johns Hopkins Medicine. https://www.hopkinsmedicine.org/health/conditions-and-diseases/pancreatic-cancer/pancreatic-cancer-vaccine-what-to-know
144. Rojas, L. A., Sethna, Z., Soares, K. C., Olcese, C., Pang, N., Patterson, E., Lihm, J., Ceglia, N., Guasp, P., Chu, A., Yu, R., Chandra, A. K., Waters, T., Ruan, J., Amisaki, M., Zebboudj, A., Odgerel, Z., Payne, G., Derhovanessian, E., ... Balachandran, V. P. (2023). Personalized RNA neoantigen vaccines stimulate T cells in pancreatic cancer. *Nature, 618*(7963), 144-150. https://doi.org/10.1038/s41586-023-06063-y

- **Oncolytic virus therapy**

    Oncolytic virus therapy is a new way to treat cancer. It uses special viruses to attack and kill cancer cells. These viruses are smart: they only target the cancer cells, not the healthy ones. Plus, they help your body's defense system, called the immune system, fight cancer even better. How do they do this? Well, they find weak spots, often found in cancer cells, and use them to destroy the cancer.[145]

    Oncolytic viruses are mostly still in the research stage. If you want to try this new treatment, you'd have to be part of a clinical trial. As of now, the FDA has approved only three types of oncolytic virus treatments. But these are only for skin cancer, called melanoma, and head and neck cancer, not pancreatic cancer. So, while oncolytic viruses are a promising idea, they aren't available for treating pancreatic cancer except in clinical trials as of summer 2023.

- **T-cell therapy**

    T-cells are like special soldier cells in our blood that help fight off harmful things like infections and cancer. What if we could take these T-cells out, make them stronger in a lab, and then put them back to fight off a serious

---

145. Nisar, M., Paracha, R. Z., Adil, S., Qureshi, S. N., & Janjua, H. A. (2022). An extensive review on preclinical and clinical trials of oncolytic viruses therapy for pancreatic cancer. *Frontiers in Oncology, 12*. https://doi.org/10.3389/fonc.2022.875188

disease like pancreatic cancer? Guess what? Scientists are actually working on this!

One group of scientists even had good results when they tested this idea on mice.[146] A hospital in Oregon said this method worked well for one of their patients.[147] Right now, clinical trials are going on to see if this clever idea can help more people.[148]

The United States is the leader in doing research on a special immunotherapy for pancreatic cancer. But it's not just the U.S.; Germany, Japan, and Italy also do a lot of work in this area. They're all trying to find better ways to treat this tough disease.[149]

---

146. Marks, R. (2022, December 15). Killing pancreatic cancer with T cells that supercharge themselves. UC San Francisco. https://www.ucsf.edu/news/2022/12/424466/killing-pancreatic-cancer-t-cells-supercharge-themselves

147. Leidner, R., Sanjuan Silva, N., Huang, H., Sprott, D., Zheng, C., Shih, Y.-P., Leung, A., Payne, R., Sutcliffe, K., Cramer, J., Rosenberg, S. A., Fox, B. A., Urba, W. J., & Tran, E. (2022). Neoantigen T-cell receptor gene therapy in pancreatic cancer. *New England Journal of Medicine, 386*(22), 2112-2119. https://doi.org/10.1056/nejmoa2119662

148. McNulty, R. (2022, March 18). Review sees potential in CAR T-cell therapy for pancreatic cancer. *The American Journal of Managed Care.* https://www.ajmc.com/view/review-sees-potential-in-car-t-cell-therapy-for-pancreatic-cancer

149. Xu, Q., Zhou, Y., Zhang, H., Li, H., Qin, H., & Wang, H. (2023, January 19). Bibliometric analysis of hotspots and frontiers of immunotherapy in pancreatic cancer. *Healthcare (Basel), 11*(3), Article 304. https://doi.org/10.3390/healthcare11030304

Consider Medications Found as a Result of Organoid Testing

As mentioned earlier, organoids can tell which of the two main chemos, FOLFIRINOX or Gemzar® + ABRAXANE® will work better for you as your first chemo.[150]

Organoids have found that some drugs already approved for other diseases can help with pancreatic cancer. For example:

- **Disulfiram (Antabuse)**

    As mentioned before, a recent discovery from testing organoids from pancreas tumors shows that a drug called disulfiram can slow down the growth of these cancer cells. Plus, it can make some cancer-fighting drugs and radiation treatment[151] work even better. Disulfiram is a medicine that helps people stop drinking alcohol. It works by making them feel very sick if they drink any alcohol. This is still a new discovery, and scientists are studying it more. If you have cancer, you could ask your cancer doctor if they think this drug could help you.[152]

---

150. Michalowski, J. (2022, November 15). How organoids can guide pancreatic cancer therapy. Cold Spring Harbor Laboratory. https://www.cshl.edu/how-organoids-can-guide-pancreatic-cancer-therapy/

151. Xu, Q., Zhou, Y., Zhang, H., Li, H., Qin, H., & Wang, H. (2023, January 19). Bibliometric analysis of hotspots and frontiers of immunotherapy in pancreatic cancer. *Healthcare (Basel), 11*(3), Article 304. https://doi.org/10.3390/healthcare11030304

152. Ahuja, N., & Coleman, J. (2012). *Patients' guide to pancreatic cancer*. Jones and Bartlett Learning. Reprinted with permission.

- **Metformin**

    This medicine for diabetes might also lower the chance of getting pancreatic cancer by about 20%. But we can't be sure yet. Scientists say we need more studies to really know if it works that way.[153]

    The impact of Metformin on people already getting treatment for pancreatic cancer is not clear-cut. A team of scientists looked at a number of studies to try and figure it out and "... found that Metformin has been shown to have augmented survival in some studies, whereas no improvement was observed in other studies."[154]

    Because the evidence isn't clear, it's a good idea to talk to your oncologist about it. Your oncologist can help you understand the latest research and how it might apply to your situation. They can also help you weigh the pros and cons of different treatment options. Remember, your doctor is there to support you and help you make the best decisions for your health.

---

153. Hu, J., Fan, H. D., Gong, J. P., & Mao, Q. S. (2023). The relationship between the use of metformin and the risk of pancreatic cancer in patients with diabetes: A systematic review and meta-analysis. *BMC Gastroenterology, 23,* Article 50. https://doi.org/10.1186/s12876-023-02671-0
154. Gyawali, M., Venkatesan, N., Ogeyingbo, O. D., Bhandari, R., Botleroo, R. A., Kareem, R., Ahmed, R., & Elshaikh, A. O. (2021, August 5). Magic of a common sugar pill in cancer: Can metformin raise survival in pancreatic cancer patients? *Cureus, 13*(8), Article e16916. https://doi.org/10.7759/cureus.16916

- **Hyaluronidase (brand name Halozyme)**

Sadly, not all early test results lead to success. For example, the drug Halozyme was created to penetrate the tough, web-like barrier surrounding pancreatic cancer (see back cover). In 2014, the FDA permitted the company to test the drug for treating pancreatic cancer that has spread to other body parts (metastatic). But by 2019, it was clear that this treatment didn't help.

Even if something looks hopeful at first, we need more research and time to know if it's actually going to work well.[155]

High-throughput screening

High-throughput is like having a fast assembly line for experiments, where many tests are conducted in a short time, providing lots of information. At UF Scripps Florida, they use advanced machines to perform this efficient testing on organoids. In their lab, they can test your pancreatic cancer cells to find what kills them with small drug-like molecules checking. They have 665,000 drugs and chemicals in stock and and can test 1,536 different kinds of drugs and mixes of drugs at a time.[156]

---

155. Hakim, N., Patel, R., Devoe, C., & Saif, M. W. (2019). Why HALO 301 failed and implications for treatment of pancreatic cancer. *Pancreas (Fairfax), 3*(1), e1-e4. https://doi.org/10.17140/POJ-3-e010
156. Spicer, T. (2023). High-throughput molecular screening center. The Herbert Wertheim UF Scripps Institute for Biomedical Innovation & Technology, Scripps Biomedical Research, University of Florida. https://scripps.ufl.edu/departments/centers-and-specialties/high-throughput-molecular-screening-center/

- **Medicines not licensed in the United States**

They even test drugs used to treat pancreatic cancer from around the world. Some of these drugs aren't allowed to be used in the United States. Some might be too risky, and others just aren't sold here for business reasons.

It's a good idea that they're testing all these different drugs, even the ones only used in other countries. Most of the time, the drugs that work best are already allowed in the U.S., but you never know. There's always a small chance they might find a drug from another country that works very well for you.[157]

If scientists discover a medicine that could really help you by testing your organoid, but it's only available in another country, you might start thinking about how to get it. One option could be to travel to that country to receive the medicine. However, before you start making any travel plans, it's crucial to have a conversation with your cancer doctor. They can offer advice on whether traveling for medicine is a wise choice. Also, it's important to thoroughly research before deciding to go abroad for treatment. Traveling for medical reasons, known as medical tourism, can be complex, challenging, and costly.

In the U.S., there's also something called the Right to Try Act. This law, passed in 2018, lets people with serious

---

157. Scripps Research. (2019). Cell-based high-throughput screening core. https://www.scripps.edu/science-and-medicine/cores-and-services/cell-based-high-throughput-screening/

illnesses try medicines that are still being tested and aren't approved yet by the FDA. These medicines have passed the first phase of testing, but they're still experimental.[158] If you're thinking about trying one of these drugs, you should definitely talk it over with your doctor. They can help you weigh the pros and cons, because these drugs can be risky since they're not fully tested yet.

Side effects of life-extending treatments versus quality of life

Knowing all your treatment options for pancreatic cancer can help you make the best choice. Doctors usually suggest standard treatments because they're proven to provide some benefit for most people. But if you're worried about side effects like feeling sick or very tired, you might want to consider other options.

By talking to a range of experts, like medical oncologists, radiation oncologists focusing on pancreatic cancer, and interventional radiologists, you'll get a well-rounded view of what is available. This way, you can pick the treatment that fits best with what you're comfortable with and need.

Balancing the side effects of life-extending treatments with quality of life is a deeply personal decision that depends on many factors. Once you pick a treatment, you should usually follow the schedule given to you and plan activities around it. But if special

---

158. FDA. (2023, January 23). *Right to try*. U.S. Food and Drug Administration. https://www.fda.gov/patients/learn-about-expanded-access-and-other-treatment-options/right-try

events like a wedding or a reunion come up, you can work with your cancer doctor to adjust your treatment schedule for those important times.

AI summarizes considerations and steps that can help:

- **Understanding Your Diagnosis and Prognosis:** Fully understand your type and stage of cancer, the expected progression, and what life-extending treatments can realistically offer. This will help you make informed decisions about your care.

- **Understanding the Side Effects of Treatment:** Learn about the possible side effects of the treatments proposed by your medical team. These can include physical effects such as fatigue, nausea, or pain, and emotional effects like depression or anxiety.

- **Assessing Your Personal Priorities:** Take the time to reflect on what's most important to you. What are your goals for the time you have left? Do you value length of life over quality of life, or vice versa? What activities or experiences do you want to have, and how might treatment side effects impact these?

- **Discussing Your Concerns with Your Medical Team:** They can provide information about the potential benefits and drawbacks of various treatments and help you make the best decision based on your situation and preferences.

- **Palliative Care and Symptom Management:** Palliative care is not just for end-of-life situations. It's about making life better for patients and their families. Palliative care doctors do this by finding and treating pain and other problems early on. This includes physical, emotional, and spiritual issues. Make sure you discuss this option with your doctor.

- **Seeking Emotional Support:** Consider seeing a therapist or counselor or joining a support group. Having open, honest conversations with your loved ones about your wishes and concerns is also important.

- **Considering Second Opinions:** If you're unsure about your treatment plan or if your priorities aren't being considered, it may be beneficial to seek a second opinion.

- **Creating an Advance Care Plan:** This includes legal documents such as a living will or durable power of attorney for health care, where you can express your wishes for end-of-life care.

- **Exploring Complementary Therapies:** Some patients find relief from side effects and stress through therapies such as acupuncture, massage, yoga, or meditation. However, always discuss these with your medical team first to ensure they won't interfere with your treatment.

Remember, there's no one right or wrong way to handle this. What matters is what feels right for you. This could depend on what you believe is important, what you like or don't like, and what your doctors and nurses say. It's okay to change your mind about your treatment if your illness gets worse or better or if what's important to you changes. Your health care team is there to help you make these tough choices.[159]

---

159. OpenAI. (2023). ChatGPT [Computer software]. Retrieved from https://www.openai.com/

Step Eleven: Monitor for Depression & Anxiety and Consider Mental Health Care

While it might sound strange, it's possible to have pancreatic cancer without constantly feeling sad. Emotional pain only makes a tough situation worse. I'm not saying you should be cheerful about having it. Instead, it's about understanding the truth of the problem and still finding happiness when you spend time with your friends, family, and special occasions.

This suggestion might be easier to understand if it comes from someone who has experienced what you're going through:

I'm not somebody who wallows in self-pity. I allowed myself time to grieve (and I did grieve because life was not the same), but then I moved on and got back to common sense. My common sense led me to the realization of "Why not me?" I had always heard that in stressful situations, people often ask "Why me?" As I pondered the journey I was on, I thought to myself—I am just a person, no better or worse than anyone else. But like everyone else on this planet, I will die someday, and in the journey comes happiness and suffering.

So, why not me? I, too, will meet suffering along my path, and this is just part of that journey. It's a humbling experience—meeting one's mortality eye-to-eye and understanding that someday I won't win the battle and hoping this wasn't that day. I remember thinking about the many blessings in my life and how good God had always been to me. I couldn't be sad, but I was wishing for more time. Isn't that what everybody wishes for at the possible end of their lifetime? And it's what we all seem to waste when it's readily available. **KH**

Here are some general strategies from AI to manage depression and anxiety while coping with pancreatic cancer:

- **Psychotherapy:** This is a vital resource for managing depression and anxiety. Cognitive-behavioral therapy (CBT—discussed in detail a little later) is particularly helpful for teaching coping skills. Other therapies like acceptance and commitment therapy (ACT) can help with the existential fears and distress that may come with a cancer diagnosis.

- **Psychiatric medication:** If your depression or anxiety symptoms are severe, medication may be necessary. Antidepressants, anti-anxiety drugs, and sleep medicines can help manage these symptoms. Always consult with your doctor before starting any new medication.

- **Support groups:** Joining a support group where people are going through a similar experience can be immensely beneficial. You can share experiences and coping strategies and find comfort in knowing you're not alone. Online platforms offer numerous support groups if you cannot find local ones.

- **Mindfulness and relaxation techniques:** Practices like mindfulness, meditation, deep breathing, and yoga can be beneficial for managing anxiety and depression. They can also improve sleep and overall mood.

- **Exercise:** As much as your condition allows, try incorporating physical activity into your daily routine. Regular exercise can boost your mood, reduce anxiety, and help you maintain your strength.

- **Healthy eating:** Eating a balanced diet is essential, especially when dealing with cancer. Certain foods may help boost your mood and energy levels.

- **Self-care:** Spend time doing activities that you enjoy and make you feel relaxed. This could be reading, painting, listening to music, or spending time in nature.

- **Stay connected:** Try to stay connected with your friends and family. It can be tempting to isolate yourself when feeling depressed and anxious, but social connections can be incredibly healing. Faith-based organizations, local support groups, chat rooms, and Facebook are examples of where invaluable support may be available. Social media is useful because several aspects of pancreatic cancer sometimes make leaving home difficult.

- **Psychosocial oncology services:** Many cancer treatment centers have specialists who help manage the emotional and social aspects of dealing with cancer. They may include psychiatrists, psychologists, and social workers experienced in helping people with the emotional aspects of cancer.

Remember, it's important to tell your health care team how you're feeling, both in your body and emotions. They can change your treatment to fit you better and give you extra help if you need it.[160]

Cognitive Behavioral Therapy (CBT) is a talk therapy where you work with a therapist to identify and change negative thoughts and behaviors. It's like having a "thought detective" who helps you understand how your thinking affects how you feel and what you do.

Of course, pancreatic cancer is a tough situation. It can sometimes make a person feel scared, sad, or even hopeless. Those feelings can affect not just their mind but also their body. They might lose sleep, not want to eat, or even have more pain because they are stressed out.

AI tells how the CBT can help:

---

160. OpenAI. (2023). ChatGPT [Computer software]. Retrieved from https://www.openai.com/

- **Changing Negative Thoughts**: Sometimes, when people are sick, they start to think very negative thoughts like "I can't handle this" or "I'm a burden." CBT helps you spot these thoughts and teaches you how to challenge them. You learn to replace them with more positive or realistic thoughts like "I'm doing the best I can" or "People do care about me."

- **Learning Coping Skills:** CBT can teach different skills like deep breathing, muscle relaxation, or how to distract yourself when you're feeling really bad. These skills can help someone deal better with pain or stress.

- **Improving Mood:** CBT can also help improve your mood by changing how you think. This is very important because when you feel better emotionally, you can also feel better physically. For example, you might have more energy or feel more up to doing things you enjoy.

- **Better Communication:** Sometimes, people with serious illnesses find it hard to talk about what they're going through. CBT can offer tips on how to communicate better with doctors, nurses, and loved ones.

- **Dealing with Symptoms:** Believe it or not, how you think can affect how you feel physically. CBT can help you experience less pain or discomfort by helping you change your mindset.

It's always good to talk with your doctor about whether CBT or any other therapy could be helpful for you. This therapy isn't a cure for pancreatic cancer, but it can help someone cope better, which can improve their quality of life.[161]

Having friends and family to talk to is very important. They can help you feel happier and less sad. People often want to be alone when they get sick with something serious like pancreatic cancer. It's okay to want alone time, especially when you're not feeling well. But being alone too much isn't good for you. You might stay away from people because you don't want to be a burden or worry about your appearance. But remember, it's good to spend time with people who care about you.

To prevent depression, it's also essential to keep your mind active, exercise regularly, and get enough sleep. However, it can be challenging to do these things when dealing with the physical symptoms of pancreatic cancer and its treatment.

Doctors might not be able to cure advanced pancreatic cancer right now, but they can definitely help with depression. Experts often say that the best way to handle depression is to take medicines that a psychiatrist gives you and also to talk things out with a psychologist. The medicines could be stimulants, antidepressants, sleeping pills, or medicines that help you feel less anxious.

---

161. OpenAI. (2023). ChatGPT [Computer software]. Retrieved from https://www.openai.com/

You can benefit from the general thoughts and prayers of others. Also, specific advice and empathy from others experiencing pancreatic cancer are very valuable. Sometimes, your friends might not know exactly what to say or what questions are all right to ask. They want to help, but they don't know how. In these situations, you can help them out by briefly telling them how you're doing medically. Then, switch over to chatting about the same things you always do. It'll be a nice break for you both. Only with your very best friends should you dive into more serious discussions.

Even though lots of people will want to stand by your side, there might be a few friends who back away. They might be scared of losing you or have some crazy idea that they could catch cancer from you. It's not your job to change their minds. Like the Beatles song says, "Let It Be."[162]

Patients often have an all-or-nothing approach to life. It is better to try to continue your normal life even if you have to modify it. If you usually have a weekly golf match, play nine holes instead or just chip and putt with your friends and go home. Same for museums and other events—leave early if you are fatigued but keep involved. Your true friends will understand.

Remember, feeling all sorts of emotions during this journey is okay. Just know you're not alone, and it's all right to lean on your support team when things get tough. That's what they're there for. Try to keep your spirits high and remember to enjoy the small moments in life. These moments can make you feel strong and help you stay hopeful.

---

162. The Beatles. (1969). *Let it be* [Album]. George Martin.

Let's talk about the power of prayer when it comes to medicine. To start, it's important to know what "faith" means. Faith means believing in someone or something, even when you can't completely prove they're real. Many people have faith that prayer can help them when they are sick, alongside regular medical treatments like medicine and surgery.

"There were prayers—so many prayers. People I didn't even know spent time praying for me. A friend had her church group knit me a prayer shawl in which each stitch represented a prayer said on my behalf." **KH**

If you have pancreatic cancer, praying and prayers of others can offer comfort and support. When you pray, you feel like you are not alone. That's really valuable.

Research demonstrates when you feel supported and less stress, your body has an easier time healing. It's like giving your body's "repair team" a boost. This is where the social support aspect comes in. When communities pray together for someone sick, that person often feels loved and supported. That can help reduce feelings of anxiety and depression, making it easier to cope with the illness.

To sum it up, prayer can be a strong partner but should not replace standard medical treatments. It offers emotional comfort and social support, which can be a big help when someone is going through a tough time with their health. Whether or not the miracle and mystery of prayer has direct healing powers is a matter of personal belief and beyond what I know for certain.

However, the comfort and support it offers are very real benefits that can help people in their journey.

I had a patient with pancreatic cancer who adopted a teddy bear poodle and named him, "Happy." She had plenty of money and staff for her and Happy, so it was a great choice. Happy truly brought her joy on tough days.

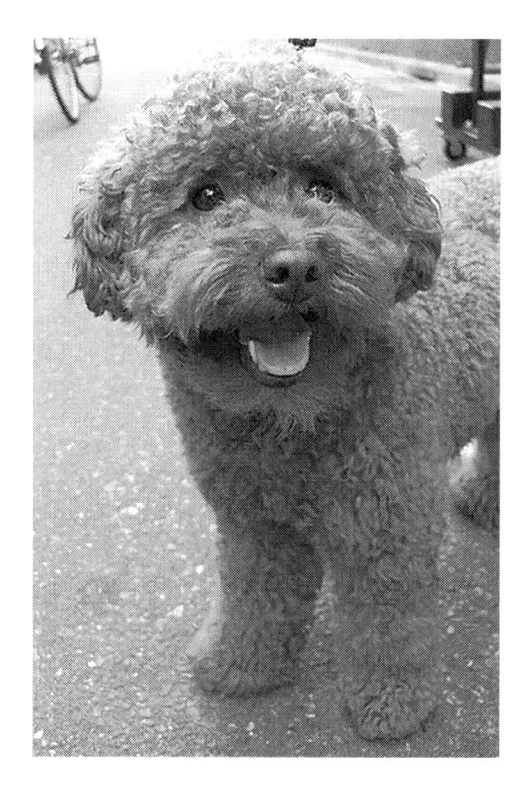

Teddy Bear Poodle[163]

---

163. Shutterstock. (n.d.). Teddy bear poodle [Photograph]. Retrieved from https://www.shutterstock.com/search/teddy-bear-poodle.

Let's turn to AI again for the pros and cons of getting a support animal, usually a dog, when you have pancreatic cancer:

Good Things:

1. **Makes You Feel Better:** A support dog can make you feel less lonely and happier. They're great for cuddles and love.

2. **Routine:** Having a dog means you have to feed them, take them out, and play with them. This routine can make you feel a bit more normal when you're dealing with being sick.

3. **Exercise:** If you're feeling up to it, a short walk with your dog can be good for you.

4. **Making Friends:** Having a dog around can help you talk to people more. It's a good way to take your mind off being sick.

5. **Less Stress:** Being around a dog can help you feel more relaxed. It's like they take away some of your worries.

6. **Unconditional Love:** Your dog will love you no matter what, and that's a great feeling to have.

7. **Distraction:** Playing with your dog or even just watching them can take your mind off the pain for a bit.

Not-So-Good Things:

1. **Cost:** Taking care of a dog costs money. You must buy food and take it to the vet.

2. **Too Much Work:** When you're sick, sometimes even small tasks can be really hard. You might not feel up to taking care of a dog.

3. **Allergies:** Some people are allergic to dogs, and that can make you feel even worse.

4. **Getting Sick:** If your immune system is weak because of treatments, you have to be careful. Dogs can carry germs. It's a good idea to talk to your doctor before getting a dog, and let them know if you already have one.

5. **Not Always Allowed:** Some hospitals and places don't let dogs in, so that can be a problem.

6. **Extra Stress:** If your dog gets sick or something happens to them, it could make you feel even worse.

7. **Treatment:** You have to make sure that taking care of your dog doesn't stop you from sticking to your medical treatments.

So, if you're thinking about getting a support animal like a dog, talk to your doctor and family to see if it's a good fit for you.[164]

---
164. OpenAI. (2023). ChatGPT [Computer software]. Retrieved from https://www.openai.com/

Step Twelve: Engage Palliative Care

According to research it's a good idea to use palliative medicine as soon as cancer treatment begins.[165] Patients do better when their symptoms and side effects are immediately taken care of.

Palliative medicine doesn't get in the way of treating pancreatic cancer. The doctors handling your palliative care will work with your oncologist and other needed specialists. The good news is that most health insurance plans cover the costs of palliative medicine.

---

165. Howie, L., & Peppercorn, J. (2013). Early palliative care in cancer treatment: Rationale, evidence and clinical implications. *Therapeutic Advances in Medical Oncology, 5*(6), 318-323. https://doi.org/10.1177/1758834013500375

Step Thirteen: Avoid Falling

(AI assisted)[166]

Introduction

For pancreatic cancer patients, the importance of avoiding falls cannot be overstated. This chapter explores why falls pose a significant risk to those with pancreatic cancer, what causes falls in older people, practical steps to prevent falls, and provides essential background information on the subject.

1. The Double Whammy of Falls for Pancreatic Cancer Patients

Falls are particularly detrimental for pancreatic cancer patients. The disease itself increases the likelihood of falling, especially at night, and simultaneously diminishes the capacity to recover from falls. Toomey and Friedman highlight the severe consequences of falls in cancer patients, including increased

---

166. OpenAI. (2023). ChatGPT [Computer software]. Retrieved from https://www.openai.com/

mortality rates.[167] This is due to both the direct impacts of the fall and the complications that arise from cancer's effects on the body. Simply put, falls can lead to severe and painful injuries or even fatalities. Therefore, patients must take all necessary precautions to prevent them.

2. Causes of Falls in the Elderly

People with pancreatic cancer need to be extra careful about falling, especially when they stand up too quickly, which is called orthostatic hypotension. This problem happens more at night. Why? Well, these patients often feel sick to their stomach, vomit, or don't feel like eating or drinking because of their cancer and the treatments they're getting. This can dehydrate them, which means their body doesn't have enough water. Also, sweating a lot at night, which can happen with this illness, worsens dehydration. Dehydration makes it harder for your body to adjust when you stand up, leading to feeling dizzy and falling. This risk is higher at night because people are sleepy and need to be slower and more careful when getting up.

The American Academy of Family Physicians outlines several other factors contributing to falls in older people. These include age-related changes like poor eyesight and hearing, medical conditions affecting strength and balance, environmental hazards such as poor lighting or loose rugs, and medication side effects. Particularly, medications for depression, sleep prob-

---

167. Toomey, A., & Friedman, L. (2014). Mortality in cancer patients after a fall-related injury: The impact of cancer spread and type. *Injury, 45*(11), 1710-1716. https://doi.org/10.1016/j.injury.2014.03.008

lems, high blood pressure, diabetes, and heart conditions can impair balance. The risk is heightened when taking four or more medications or after recent changes in medication.[168]

3. Strategies to Avoid Falls

Having a nurse or an aide around, especially at night, can really help. They can make sure the person with pancreatic cancer doesn't get up too fast and can be there to support them if they feel dizzy. This help can prevent falls, keeping the patient safer.

To mitigate the risk of falls, the 2010 AGS and BGS guidelines recommend multifactorial interventions, with the strongest evidence supporting home modifications and exercise. Adjusting medications, managing postural hypotension, and addressing foot problems and footwear are also advised. Practical steps include removing tripping hazards, securing (using double-sided tape) or removing rugs, ensuring easy access to frequently used items, installing grab bars in bathrooms, using non-slip mats, enhancing home lighting, and wearing well-fitting shoes. These measures can significantly reduce the risk of falls and their associated injuries.[169]

---

168. American Academy of Family Physicians. (2000, April 1). What causes falls in the elderly? How can I prevent a fall? *American Family Physician.* https://www.aafp.org/pubs/afp/issues/2000/0401/p2173.html
169. Al-Aama, T. (2011). Falls in the elderly: Spectrum and prevention. *Canadian Family Physician, 57*(7), 771-776. https://www.ncbi.nlm.nih.gov/pmc/articles/PMC3135440/

In addition to the measures mentioned, pancreatic cancer patients should focus on:

1. **Pausing Upon Standing:** Take a moment to stand still after getting up. This pause allows the blood pressure to adjust.

2. **Adequate Hydration:** Maintaining hydration is crucial for blood pressure stability.

3. **Coasting Technique:** Lightly placing a hand on furniture and countertops for support while moving around.

Background Information on Falls Among the Elderly

Falls are a common and serious issue among older adults. The Centers for Disease Control and Prevention reports that annually, about 36 million falls occur among older adults, leading to over 32,000 deaths and 3 million emergency department treatments. One in five falls causes significant injuries, such as broken bones or head injuries. Hip fractures are particularly common, with more than 95% resulting from falls, predominantly sideways falls. Women are more susceptible to falls and account for three-quarters of all hip fractures.[170]

---

170. Centers for Disease Control and Prevention. (2023, March 24). Keep on your feet—preventing older adult falls. Retrieved from https://www.cdc.gov/injury/features/older-adult-falls/index.html

Patient Education

Understanding how our body functions normally and what changes occur in certain conditions like pancreatic cancer, especially in older people, is essential. Let's start by explaining the basics of blood circulation and then discuss the specific issue of orthostatic hypotension, a common risk for elderly patients, especially those with health conditions like pancreatic cancer:

1. **Normal Body Function and Blood Circulation:** About 1¼ to 1½ gallons of blood circulate continuously in a healthy body. This blood, which is akin to saltwater with proteins and tiny iron particles, flows effortlessly throughout the body. When someone lies down, their blood evenly distributes across the body, maintaining a level balance with the heart. This seamless flow ensures that all body parts, from the toes to the brain, receive adequate blood supply.

2. **Changes from Lying to Standing:** However, this equilibrium is challenged when a person stands up. Standing up introduces a fight against gravity, as gravity naturally pulls the blood towards the lower parts of the body, like the feet and legs. To counter this, our body employs a smart mechanism. Special nerves called 'baroreceptors', which monitor blood pressure, sense this change in position. In response, the blood vessels in the legs constrict or narrow, effectively pushing the blood upwards toward the brain and upper body. This quick adaptation by the body helps

maintain a steady blood flow and pressure even when the body's position changes.[171]

3. **Elderly and Pancreatic Cancer Patients:** In elderly individuals, and more so in those with conditions like pancreatic cancer, this system may not work as efficiently. As we age, these baroreceptors become less sensitive and our blood vessels are respond slower and not as well to standing. This reduced sensitivity can lead to orthostatic hypotension, a condition where blood pressure falls significantly when moving from a lying or sitting position to standing. This drop in blood pressure can cause dizziness due to reduced blood flow to the brain, increasing the risk of falling.

Conclusion

For pancreatic cancer patients, preventing falls is critical to their care. Understanding the causes of falls and implementing effective prevention strategies can greatly enhance their safety and well-being. A nurse or health aide's involvement, especially at night, can provide additional support in preventing falls, thereby reducing the risk of severe injuries or complications.

---

171. Brodkey, F. D., & Dugdale, D. C. (2023). Aging changes in the heart and blood vessels. In *MedlinePlus Medical Encyclopedia*. Retrieved from https://medlineplus.gov/ency/article/004006.htm

Step Fourteen: Use Home Nursing and Other Supportive Services

If you have pancreatic cancer, figuring out who should take care of you can be hard. You might think your family can help, and they can in many ways. But sometimes, professionals might be the better choice. Here's why:

- **More Comfort with Less Awkwardness**

    Let's be honest: being bathed or helped in the bathroom by your adult kids or even your spouse can be weird for you and them. Nurses do this all the time and know how to make it less awkward.

- **Expert Care**

    At times, family members may find it hard to keep up with the schedule of medicines and make sure they're taken when they're supposed to be. Medicines might also have side effects that can make you feel unwell or uncomfortable in several ways. Some of these side effects are small and you might just need to adjust to them, but some are serious and require quick action. It's very important to be able to recognize the serious side effects, know how to respond to them, and keep a record of all side effects to talk about with your doctor later.

Pancreatic cancer and its treatments can cause you to feel nauseous, have accidents, or experience pain. Professional nurses know exactly how to deal with these challenging issues. They can help and advise on how to manage these side effects, which can make going through treatment a little bit easier.

- **They're Used to It**

    Taking care of someone with pancreatic cancer is a big job and can be really exhausting for family members, especially if they're doing it all by themselves for a long time. Luckily, there are professional home health care workers who are trained specifically for this kind of work. They can step in to help for a few days, giving your family a break. This help is called respite care, and it's all about offering relief to families in need. Or they can provide on-going care.

    These professionals can help with different caregiving tasks. They can assist with daily activities like feeding and bathing, take care of things during the night, or even handle all the tasks that need to be done. The good news is, there are usually several professionals available, so they can take turns helping out. This means there's always someone there rested and ready to support you, which can make everyone feel less stressed and more taken care of.

- **Family Can Be There in Other Ways**

  When you have a nurse or therapist, your family can focus on giving you love and emotional support. They can also make sure the professionals are doing a good job.

- **Downsides**

  Using professional home health care has some disadvantages. One downside is that you have less privacy because having professionals in your home means you're not alone as much. Another downside is the cost, as home care can become quite expensive over time.

- **Money Matters and Family Roles:**

  1. **Cost:** Check what your health and long-term care insurance covers because some of this can get pricey.

  2. **Family Income:** If a family member has to quit their job or work less to help you, that's tough on money.

  3. **Best Job for Family Members:** They're often best at giving emotional support and checking on the home health pros. They can help in an emergency, too.

Despite these issues, professional home care can be a good option. It's important to talk with your family and your doctor to make the best choice for your situation.

- **Different Types of Home Care (these are from least to most expensive):**

    1. **Home Health Aide:** Helps with simple activities like eating and bathing.

    2. **Occupational Therapy:** Teaches you new ways to do daily tasks.

    3. **Physical Therapy:** Helps you get stronger and move better.

    4. **LPN (Licensed Practical Nurse):** Helps with medicines and simple nursing tasks.

    5. **RN (Registered Nurse):** Takes care of more complex health needs.

    6. **Specialized Nurses:** Know a lot about specific problems like cancer.

- **How to Hire Home Health Care Professionals**

When you get nursing help at your home, it should be customized to fit your needs. Even if you believe you don't need help during the night, you might be mistaken. In the last chapter, we talked about how easy it is to fall and how having a night nurse or aide can prevent this. Also, people with pancreatic cancer often sweat a lot while sleeping. They might need assistance with sponge baths or changing their clothes, possibly more than once during the night. Remember, you can always adjust the services based on what you need and can pay for.

1. **Nursing agencies:** If you want to hire a nurse to help you at home, the easiest way is to use a nursing agency. These agencies find good nurses for you. They make sure the nurses are trustworthy and manage their work schedules. But this service is not cheap. They usually charge a lot more than the nurses get paid. If you want a RN to be with you all day and all night for a whole year, it could cost around $500,000 if you use an agency. ($$$$).

2. **Nursing registries:** Nursing registries are like organized lists of nurses. They are not as picky regarding education and experience as agencies when it comes to choosing nurses. You can often save money by hiring nurses from a registry instead of from an agency ($$$+).

3. **Direct hiring:** If you need a nurse to help at home, you might think about hiring a nurse yourself instead

of going through an agency. It could save you some money. But keep in mind it's a lot of work! Since there are 168 hours in a week, you'll need four or five nurses if you need someone 24/7.

Hiring a nurse is more than just finding someone good at taking care of people. You also have to look into their past to make sure they're trustworthy. You should consider testing them to make sure they're not using illegal or recreational drugs.

Remember, you'll be the one paying them. On top of their pay, keeping up with taxes and other job-related paperwork can take a lot of time and cost extra money. One of the biggest things to think about is if a home health worker gets hurt while at your house, you might need to pay for their injuries. That's why having worker's compensation insurance is a smart move.

You must check that they have the right nursing license. Also, you'll need to keep track of when their license needs to be renewed.

- **Insurance Coverage for Home Health Care (AI assisted):**

    1. **Medicare** is for people 65 and older or with certain disabilities. It usually covers short-term home health care. You must have a doctor say you need it. How to find out what's covered and apply:

A. Talk to your doctor. They need to write an order for home health care.

B. Visit the Medicare website or call to see what's covered.

C. Pick a Medicare-approved home health agency to get your services.

2. **Medicaid** helps low-income people. What it covers for home health care can be different depending on your state. How to find out what's covered and apply:

A. Contact your state's Medicaid office to see what they cover.

B. You usually need a doctor to say that you need home care.

C. Fill out the needed forms and wait to hear back.

3. **Commercial Plans** are insurance plans that you or your job pays for. Coverage for home health care varies a lot from plan to plan. Some don't cover home health care while others provide generous benefits. How to find out what's covered and apply:

A. Check your insurance policy or call customer service.

B. Have your doctor write an order for home health care.

C. Submit the order and any other paperwork your insurance asks for.

4. **Long-Term Care Insurance:** is often the best for home health care that lasts a long time. But you have to buy this before you need the care. How to find out what's covered and apply:

   A. Read your policy or talk to the company to see what is covered.

   B. Have a doctor say you need long-term home care.

   C. Send this info to the insurance company and wait for approval.

   Remember, it's always good to double-check what's covered to avoid surprise bills.[172]

Care by Family Members

If your family is going to care for you, they will need to know several important concepts. While I cannot provide comprehensive instructions here, important skills include the following:

- Helping you avoid aspiration into your lungs when eating and especially, vomiting.

---

[172]. OpenAI. (2023). ChatGPT [Computer software]. Retrieved from https://www.openai.com/

- Accurately taking your temperature.

- Moving you in bed from side to side to avoid pressure ulcers.

- Helping you avoid dehydration even if you are nauseated.

- Knowing when to use "as needed" medications.

- Knowing the signs and symptoms that indicate a need to call 911 and then your doctor. They include the following:

    1. Difficulty awakening

    2. Acute confusion as compared to hours earlier.

    3. Fever higher than a number set by the doctor.

    4. Vomiting blood

    5. Shortness of breath

    6. Chest pain

Step Fifteen: Living with Pancreatic Cancer

Managing Day-to-Day Symptoms and Side Effects

Always talk to your doctor or nurse about any side effects—they're there to help you!

- **Nausea and Vomiting:**

    Chemotherapy is a usual way to treat pancreatic cancer, but it can make you sick and throw up a lot. If you have this problem, ask your doctor for medicine to help with the nausea. Eating smaller meals more often instead of three big ones can also help. Drink lots of water and other drinks and stay away from very spicy or greasy food.

- **Fatigue:**

    Feeling very tired is normal when you're getting treatment for cancer. To help with this, make sure to rest a lot. But also do some light exercise like walking or easy yoga, because it can help you feel more energetic. Eating healthy food and drinking plenty of liquids can also make you feel better.

- **Pain:**

    Pancreatic cancer or the treatment can sometimes hurt. If you're in pain, your doctor can give you medicine to help. Make sure you take it just like your doctor says and tell them if it doesn't work well. Some people feel better with relaxation exercises, like taking deep breaths or meditating, to help with the pain.

- **Weight loss and Appetite Changes:**

    You might lose weight and/or not want to eat when you have pancreatic cancer. To keep your weight up, try eating small meals often during the day. Eat foods with lots of protein, like eggs, milk products, or meats that aren't too fatty. Your doctor might also say you should see a person who knows a lot about food, a dietitian, to help you figure out what to eat.

From AI, "Seek out dietary advice and nutrition counseling. Managing diet can be a key part of managing pancreatic cancer and treatment side effects."[173]

- **Digestive Issues:**

The pancreas is an organ that helps break down food, so when you have pancreatic cancer, you may have diarrhea or constipation. If you have these problems, your doctor might suggest taking medicine, eating different foods, or trying other things to make you feel better.

Work

Per AI:

Working can help someone deal with pancreatic cancer in a few different ways:

1. **Feeling Purposeful and Normal:** Having a job can make you feel like you have a reason to get up in the morning. It can also help you have a regular schedule and feel more normal. This is very good for your mind, especially if you're going through a tough time with your health.

---
173. OpenAI. (2023). ChatGPT [Computer software]. Retrieved from https://www.openai.com/

2. **Making and Keeping Friends at Work:** Staying at your job can give you chances to talk to other people and make friends. This can help you feel less alone and sad, which might happen when you find out you have cancer.

3. **Taking Your Mind Off Things:** Having a job can help you stop thinking about the stress and worry that comes with having cancer. It can take your mind off your illness.

4. **Financial Support:** Keeping your job can help you have enough money to pay for things, which is important because cancer and its treatment can be very expensive.

Balancing work/productivity with taking care of yourself and managing cancer symptoms and their treatments is important. Here are some ideas for managing work or other activities while living with pancreatic cancer:

1. **Prioritize tasks:** Decide which tasks are most important and do them when you have the most energy. Remember that it's okay to put some things off for another time or ask for help when needed.

2. **Listen to your body:** If you're tired or unwell, take a break or rest when needed. Pay attention to how your body responds to different activities and adjust your schedule accordingly.

3. **Communicate with others:** Let your coworkers, boss, or friends know about your condition and any limitations you might have. They may be more understanding and supportive if they know what you're going through.

4. **Set realistic goals:** Be realistic about what you can achieve and set achievable goals. If you used to be able to finish a project in a day, you might now need two or three days. That's okay!

5. **Consider a flexible schedule:** If you're working, talk to your employer about flexible working hours or telecommuting options. This way, you can work during the times you feel best and take breaks when you need them.

6. **Ask for help:** It's okay to ask for help when you need it. Whether it's asking a coworker to cover for you or asking a friend to help you with household tasks, you don't have to do everything on your own.

7. **Take care of your physical and mental well-being:** Eat nutritious food, get some exercise, and try to get enough sleep. Again, consider joining a support group or talking to a therapist to help you cope with the emotional challenges of dealing with pancreatic cancer.

It's important to strike a balance between staying productive and taking care of yourself. Remember that you're not alone in this journey, and it's okay to lean on others for support when you need it.[174]

Travel

"Once I got past that difficult first six months, I began traveling with my family. I found that cruises were best for me as my bed was always nearby when I was feeling unwell." **JG**

Thoughts from AI:

Traveling is often a fun way to explore new places and cultures, and it can also be a helpful way to cope with difficult experiences, like dealing with pancreatic cancer. Even if you have been diagnosed with pancreatic cancer, traveling can still be an option for you as long as you make sure to prioritize your health and balance your travel plans with your treatment schedule and the need for extra rest.

Here are a few ways traveling can help someone with pancreatic cancer:

1. **New experiences:** Traveling to new places and experiencing new cultures can take your mind off the stress and challenges of a cancer diagnosis.

---

174. OpenAI. (2023). ChatGPT [Computer software]. Retrieved from https://www.openai.com/

2. **Relaxation:** Sometimes, you only need a change of scenery to help you relax and recharge. Traveling to a serene and peaceful destination can provide a much-needed break from the hustle and bustle of daily life.

3. **Strengthening relationships:** Traveling with loved ones can help strengthen relationships and create lasting memories, even in challenging times.

If you have pancreatic cancer and are considering traveling, it's important to consider the following:

1. **Consult your health care team:** Before making any travel plans, talk to your health care team about your specific needs and the logistics of traveling. They can provide advice on how to balance treatment schedules and travel plans and whether it's safe for you to travel.

2. **Plan for extra rest:** Traveling can be exhausting for anyone, but especially for someone with cancer. Make sure to build in time for rest and relaxation in your travel plans, and adjust your plans as needed based on how you feel.

3. **Consider the destination:** Some destinations may be more suitable than others for someone with pancreatic cancer. For example, it may be easier to travel to places with good health care facilities or where you have friends or family who can help if needed.

4. **Prepare for potential symptoms:** Pancreatic cancer and its treatment can cause a range of symptoms, such as pain or fatigue. Be prepared to manage these symptoms while traveling, and make sure you have any medications or other supplies you might need.

5. **Travel insurance:** Make sure you have travel insurance that covers your specific needs and that you understand any limitations or restrictions related to pre-existing conditions.

Traveling can be a great way to feel better when you're dealing with pancreatic cancer. But remember, staying healthy is the most important thing. You'll need to plan your trip carefully, so it fits with your medical treatments and allows you time to rest. With good planning, you can still have an awesome trip and make memories that will last a lifetime.[175]

Doing Your Own Research

Randomized/Peer-Reviewed Studies Are the Best

If you or someone you know has been diagnosed with pancreatic cancer, doing your own research can be a powerful tool in understanding the disease and making informed choices. With so much information out there, knowing where to look and what to trust is important. Medical experts are the best source

---

175. OpenAI. (2023). ChatGPT [Computer software]. Retrieved from https://www.openai.com/

of advice, but having extra knowledge can help you feel more in control and make better decisions. The following paragraphs will guide you through understanding different kinds of medical studies, how to read scientific articles, and how to spot false or misleading information. We'll also touch on how technology like AI can assist you and why some studies, like those on animals, will probably take too long to impact your care.

Reading a whole science article might feel like a lot. But don't worry! You can get the main ideas by reading the abstract, introduction, and summary. AI adds a few more details:

I'll give you some extra details randomized controlled trials. These are the best for finding out if a treatment really works. Here's why:

- **Randomization:** In RCTs, they put people in the treatment or control group by chance. This helps make sure the results are because of the treatment and not something else.

- **Controlled:** Most RCTs have a control group that gets a fake treatment (placebo) and/or the usual treatment. The treatment group gets the new treatment. Scientists can see if the new treatment is better by comparing these groups.

- **Blinding:** RCTs often use blinding, where the people in the study, the researchers, or both, only know who's getting the new treatment at the end. This helps make the results more believable.

- **Reproducibility:** RCTs are designed so other scientists can repeat the same study and check the results.

But remember, RCTs aren't the only good science studies. Others, like cohort studies, case-control studies, and observational studies, can give important information, too. Systematic reviews and meta-analyses, which look at many studies together, can also give important information.[176]

Online, Newspaper, and Magazine Articles

Almost always, these articles come from just one published paper. If the study doesn't say where it came from, you can usually find it with a quick online search.

Here are a few important things to remember when reading news articles:

- Don't pay attention to advertisements or self-promotion. Cancer treatments that work do not need to be advertised.

- When you're looking for trustworthy information, especially about medical topics, focus on reports that share new findings from medical journals or conferences. If an article doesn't come from these reliable sources, it's probably not something you should trust.

---

[176]. OpenAI. (2023). ChatGPT [Computer software]. Retrieved from https://www.openai.com/

Beware of Predatory Journals

A predatory journal is a fake science magazine that tricks the public. Authors pay to publish their article. Predatory journals don't do a good job of checking the quality of the articles or might not check them at all. It's a shady business that pretends to be a real scientific publication.[177]

AI tells us that if you're not an expert, spotting misleading information in a bad or "predatory" journal might be tricky. But don't worry, there are some signs you can look for:

- **Look for Errors:** This might seem simple, but a lot of bad papers have mistakes like spelling errors and bad grammar. Good science writing should be clear and correct.

- **Does It Sound Too Good to Be True?** If the paper claims to solve a major problem easily, be suspicious. Almost always, real science is a slow process with small steps forward, not giant leaps.

- **Who Wrote It?** Look at who the authors are. If they're from a reputable institution or university, the paper might be trustworthy. If you can't find any information about the authors, that's a bad sign.

- **Who Checked It?** Other experts check real science before it gets published. This is called "peer review." Be careful if

---

177. OpenAI. (2023). ChatGPT [Computer software]. Retrieved from https://www.openai.com/

the paper doesn't mention who reviewed it or if the review took only a few days.

- **Check the Data:** Good papers should have lots of data and facts to back up what they're saying. If a paper makes a lot of claims but doesn't give any proof, be suspicious.

- **Do Other Experts Agree?** If other experts mention the paper and agree with it, it's a good sign. If nobody else is talking about it or they disagree, be careful.

Remember, just because something is published, it doesn't mean it's true. Always be skeptical and check the facts. If you're not sure, you can always ask your doctor or other knowledgeable person for help.[178]

Using Artificial Intelligence

Funny... AI can help us learn to use AI. For someone diagnosed with pancreatic cancer, finding the best doctors and treatments is important. AI, again short for artificial intelligence, can help with this. It's like a super-smart computer that can quickly sort through a ton of information.

Here's how AI can help:

---

178. OpenAI. (2023). ChatGPT [Computer software]. Retrieved from https://www.openai.com/

- **Finding the Best Doctors:** AI can look through a lot of data about doctors. It can find doctors specializing in treating pancreatic cancer and those with a lot of experience. AI can also read reviews from other patients.

- **Understanding Treatments:** AI can help you understand different treatments for pancreatic cancer. It can tell you about the latest research, explain what treatments do, and even tell you about possible side effects.

- **Connecting with Others:** Some types of AI can help connect you with other people who have pancreatic cancer. You can learn from their experiences and get support.[179]

Why should you use AI? There are three big reasons:

- **Save Time:** AI can look through information really quickly. It would take you much longer to find all that info yourself.

- **Stay Updated:** AI can help you stay up to date. In the world of medicine, new things are discovered all the time. AI can help you keep track of the latest news and research.

- **Be Informed:** The more you know, the better choices you can make. Using AI can help you learn much about your disease, doctors, and treatment options.

---

179. OpenAI. (2023). ChatGPT [Computer software]. Retrieved from https://www.openai.com/

Remember, AI is a tool to help you, but it's not perfect. Always talk to your doctor about what you find. They can help you understand the information and make the best choices for you.[180]

Mouse Studies Are Not Very Reliable and Take a Long Time to Possibly Affect Your Medical Treatment

For pancreatic cancer, you want the best treatment and doctors. You might learn about interesting studies where scientists are trying out new treatments on animals; for example, mice. These animal studies are very important because they help scientists understand diseases better.

But here's the catch: what works for a mouse, or another animal, might not work for a human. And it takes a really long time, like years, to take something that helped a mouse and make it safe and effective for people. If you're looking for a treatment you can use sooner, it's smarter to look at options already being tested on humans.

So, talk to your doctors about treatments that have been proven to work in people. This way, you're focusing on choices that are closer to being available for you and can help you get better faster.

---

180. OpenAI. (2023). ChatGPT [Computer software]. Retrieved from https://www.openai.com/

Stay Organized

Staying organized is really important when learning about pancreatic cancer, especially during talks with your doctor. They'll only give you so much time and answer a few well-thought-out questions. Write a list of your questions and remember to take it with you.

You might find a lot of different pieces of information, like new treatment methods, alternative therapies, suggested doctors and hospitals, ways to reduce side effects, and advice on diets and supplements. To make sure you remember everything and can find it again later, it's a good idea to keep track of where each piece of information comes from.

For example, if you find a helpful piece of information in a video, write down the web address (URL) of the video and the time when the important information is mentioned. If you learn something from a book or a person, make a note of the book's title or the person's name. If you find information on a website, write down the website's address. Another method is to copy/paste the URL and email it to yourself. Keep all this information together in a place where you can easily find it again.

AI gives us more about each type of information you might want to look for:

- **New treatments:** Medicine keeps getting better. Doctors and scientists always look for new ways to help people with pancreatic cancer. Watching for any news or updates about these new treatments is a good idea.

- **Alternative treatments:** Besides the usual medical treatments, there are alternative therapies that some people find helpful. These include herbal medicine, acupuncture, or yoga. It's important to check with your doctor before trying these, but you can still collect information about them.

- **Recommended doctors and hospitals:** Different doctors and hospitals have different specialties. Some might be particularly good at treating pancreatic cancer. If you hear about a doctor or a hospital that's highly recommended, write down their name and contact information.

- **Ways to minimize side effects:** Treatments for pancreatic cancer can sometimes have side effects. These might include feeling tired, losing weight, or having an upset stomach. But there are often ways to lessen these side effects, like changing your diet or taking certain medications. If you learn any tips for dealing with side effects, write them down. Before you take anything, even if it's just an over-the-counter medicine, check with your doctor or nurse.

- **Diets and Supplements:** What you eat can make a difference in how you feel when you're being treated for pancreatic cancer. Certain foods or dietary supplements might be recommended to help your body stay strong and deal with the effects of treatment. Again, for emphasis, before you take anything, even if it's just a vitamin or supplement, check with your doctor or nurse. If you learn about any foods, diets, or supplements suggested for people with pancreatic cancer, note them.

Remember, it's essential to keep everything organized and easy to find. That way, you'll be able to find and refer to the information whenever you need.[181]

Suggested Web Searches:

- Pathology second opinion

- Pancreatic cancer radiology second opinion

- Best hospitals for cancer

- Remote second opinion cancer

- Pancreatic cancer organoid clinical research

- Physician license lookup (see state websites in Appendix A)

Videos:

- https://youtu.be/YmsR_Vmom8o (Nutrition—time range 3:43 to 4:24)

---

181. OpenAI. (2023). ChatGPT [Computer software]. Retrieved from https://www.openai.com/

- https://youtu.be/DH9m-4bRYOc (About organoids, beginning at the two-minute mark for a couple of minutes—beyond then it becomes confusingly detailed)

Participating in Clinical Trials

AI:

Clinical trials are studies done with people to test a new medical treatment, surgery, or behavior change. These studies are how scientists figure out if a new drug, diet, or medical tool is safe and works well in people. These trials can also show what treatments are best for certain diseases or groups of people. AI lists the pros and cons for your participation:

Pros:

1. **Access to new treatments:** Being in a clinical trial lets you try new treatments that other people can't get yet. This could be good if other treatments haven't worked for you.

2. **Close Monitoring:** In a clinical trial, doctors and nurses watch your health closely. You get checked up on more often, and the team carefully monitors how you're doing.

3. **Helping others:** The info from clinical trials can help people in the future. Your participation might help find a new treatment that could help lots of people.

Cons:

1. **Uncertain outcomes:** The new treatments in clinical trials may not always be better than, or even as good as, regular treatments. They might not work for you, even if they work for others.

2. **Side effects:** All treatments can have side effects. Since the treatments in clinical trials are new, doctors might still need to learn all the side effects. Some might be uncomfortable, serious, or even dangerous.

3. **Time and commitment:** Being in a clinical trial can take up a lot of time. You might have more doctor visits, treatments, hospital stays, or confusing medicine schedules.

4. **Placebo:** In randomized clinical trials, some people get a placebo, which are pills that do not contain drugs. Amazingly, there is some benefit called the placebo effect.[182]

However, the placebo effect is not as large as some think. "... placebos are sometimes associated with improved control of symptoms such as pain and appetite but rarely with positive tumor response. Substantial improvements in symptoms and quality of life are unlikely to be due to placebo effects."[183]

---

182. OpenAI. (2023). ChatGPT [Computer software]. Retrieved from https://www.openai.com/
183. Chvetzoff, G., & Tannock, I. F. (2003, January 1). Placebo effects in oncology. *Journal of the National Cancer Institute, 95*(1), 19-29. https://doi.org/10.1093/jnci/95.1.19

- **How to Apply for Clinical Trials:**

In the US, your doctor can help you find clinical trials that could be good for you. They can explain the trial, what to expect, and help you apply. You can also look for clinical trials yourself. Websites like ClinicalTrials.gov have lists of trials that are happening now. Make sure to talk to your health care provider before you apply.

If you're looking for more treatment options, you might think about joining clinical trials in other countries. These are called international clinical trials, and they can give you more choices for getting better. But joining trials in another country isn't as simple as it sounds. You'll have to think about things like speaking a different language, traveling there, and understanding how health care works in that country.

Also, be careful. Just because getting into a clinical trial in Australia might be easier doesn't mean it's always a good idea. Sometimes, treatments that look good at first don't end up working well. So, if you're thinking about going to another country for treatment, make sure to talk it over really well with your doctors. You don't want to rush into something that might not help you, just because you're eager to find a cure.

Johns Hopkins Medicine suggests "a list of questions that you should consider asking to help guide you in decision-making and fact-finding about clinical trials:"[184]

---

184. Ahuja, N., & Coleman, J. (2012). *Patients' guide to pancreatic cancer.* Jones & Bartlett Learning. Reprinted with permission.

- What is the purpose of the study?

- How many people will be included in the study?

- What does the study involve?

- What kind of tests and treatment will I have?

- How are treatments given and what side effects might I expect?

- What are the risks and benefits of each protocol?

- What alternatives do I have to participating in the study?

- How long will the study last?

- What type of long-term follow-up care is provided for those who participate?

- Will I incur any costs?

- Will my insurance company pay for part of this?

- When will the results be known?[185]

AI says clinical trials are important tests that help scientists figure out if a medicine or treatment works. No

---

185. Ahuja, N., & Coleman, J. (2012). *Patients' guide to pancreatic cancer.* Jones & Bartlett Learning. Reprinted with permission.

matter where a trial happens—in the U.S. or another country—it must be watched closely to make sure it's safe and follows ethical rules.

In the United States, special groups called "Institutional Review Boards" act like referees. The members usually consist of doctors, researchers, ethics experts, lawyers and even a member from the general public. They make sure the rules are followed, even if those rules are strict. For example, if you're going to be part of a medical test, you usually need to have tried at least two chemotherapy treatments that didn't work for you. And remember, if you ever feel uncomfortable or change your mind, you can leave a clinical trial whenever you want, for any reason.[186]

Healthy Living

Living a healthy lifestyle can definitely help someone who has pancreatic cancer. You might be surprised that consistently getting enough and good quality sleep is my first and most important recommendation. When you don't get enough sleep, other things in your life can get worse. It's hard to work out when you're sleepy. Also, if you're tired, you might eat more sugary foods or carbs for a quick energy boost. Plus, you might drink a lot of caffeine to feel more alert.

AI helps us understand what healthy living means:

---

186. OpenAI. (2023). ChatGPT [Computer software]. Retrieved from https://www.openai.com/

Adequate sleep

When you have pancreatic cancer, you might feel very tired and yet find it hard to sleep. This could be because of the cancer itself, the stress it brings, and the side effects of your medicine. You may need to sleep more than usual because the cancer and its treatment can make you super tired.

Sleep is very important, just like food and water. When we sleep, our bodies and brains rest and recharge. But what if you have pancreatic cancer and can't sleep well? This problem is called insomnia, which means you have trouble falling asleep or staying asleep.

Why is sleep so important when fighting pancreatic cancer?

- Sleep helps your body heal. When you're sick, your body is working extra hard. Without enough sleep, your body might not have enough energy to fight the disease.

- Sleep helps your brain. It can help you think clearly, make good choices, and feel less sad or worried.

What can you do if pancreatic cancer causes insomnia?

- If you're uncomfortable because of cancer or treatment side effects, ask your doctor about pain relief or other options.

- If you're stressed or worried, try deep breathing, meditation, or talking to a counselor.

- To have good sleep habits, try to go to bed and get up at the same time every day. Make sure your bedroom is dark and quiet. Also, avoid having things like coffee or spending time on your TV, phone, or computer right before bed. These can make it harder to fall asleep.

If you're tired, taking short naps during the day is okay, but not too much because it could make it harder to sleep at night. Talk to your doctor if you're very tired, as it could be a sign of something else or that your treatment needs adjustment. They might suggest exercises or changes in your diet.

In conclusion, sleep is a powerful tool when fighting pancreatic cancer. Even though insomnia can be common, there are many ways to deal with it. By focusing on sleep and managing insomnia, people with pancreatic cancer can give their bodies and minds the best chance to heal and fight the disease. Remember to listen to your body and ask your medical team for help if you need it.[187]

Diet

Eating the right foods can give your body the nutrients it needs to stay strong. For someone with pancreatic cancer, it's important to eat a balanced diet with plenty of fruits, vegetables, and proteins. These foods can help your body fight off sickness and can also help you keep your strength up.

---

187. OpenAI. (2023). ChatGPT [Computer software]. Retrieved from https://www.openai.com/

You should consider some important points about what to eat when it comes to pancreatic cancer:

- **Pancreatic Enzymes:** Sometimes, people with pancreatic cancer don't have enough pancreatic enzymes that help digest food. Luckily, these can be replaced with supplements. Prescription pancreatic enzymes are recommended because they are usually better quality, and you take them under your doctor's direction.[188]

- **Sugar Debate:** There is a debate about whether people with pancreatic cancer should any eat sugar, especially "free sugars." Free sugars are added to foods and drinks or found naturally in fruit juices and maple syrup. Some people think these sugars might harm those with pancreatic cancer, while others disagree. This is a complex topic with no final answer. Speaking to your doctor or dietitian for advice that suits your health needs is always a good idea.

- **Sugar and Cancer:** It's often said that sugar feeds cancer cells. But it's more complex than that. Sugar is a simple form of carbohydrate, and carbs give us energy. Carbs are found in foods like bread, pasta, fruits, and sweets. Cancer cells need glucose (a type of sugar) to grow like all our cells do. But cancer cells might use more glucose because they're more active.

---

188. Pancreatic Cancer Action Network. (2023, August 1). Pancreatic enzymes. Retrieved from https://pancan.org/facing-pancreatic-cancer/living-with-pancreatic-cancer/diet-and-nutrition/pancreatic-enzymes/

Eating more carbs doesn't directly "feed" cancer cells, as our body controls our glucose levels. There is some evidence that a high-sugar diet might be linked to getting pancreatic cancer, but more research is needed. If you have pancreatic cancer, it's important to have a balanced diet. Too much sugar isn't good for anyone, but cutting out all sugar and carbs isn't going to cure pancreatic cancer. Talk to a doctor or dietitian for the best advice.[189]

Moderate exercise

An article that looked at many studies about people with breast and colon cancer discovered that walking "has a huge impact on survival."[190] While this study was not about those with pancreatic cancer, it is reasonable to assume that walking would be great for you also.

Physical activity can make you feel better and give you more strength and energy. When you move, it helps blood flow, bringing oxygen and nutrients to your whole body, including sick parts. Exercise also releases chemicals in your brain that make you happy and can help with side effects of cancer treatment, like tiredness and feeling sick. It can also help you sleep better, eat more, and feel better overall.

---

189. OpenAI. (2023). ChatGPT [Computer software]. Retrieved from https://www.openai.com/
190. Borland, S. (2017). Daily 30-minute walk may slash cancer deaths by half: Studies find regular exercise has a huge impact on survival by slowing tumour growth. *Daily Mail.* http://www.dailymail.co.uk/news/article-4575268/Daily-30-minute-walk-slash-cancer-deaths-half.html

But if you have pancreatic cancer, listen to your body. If you're very tired or sick, it might not be a good day for any exercise, certainly not hard exercise. Doing too much can make you tired, worsen your symptoms, or cause injury. Walking for just a few minutes once or twice a day might be enough. If you feel good, try walking for 30-45 minutes every day. On other days, add light weights or use exercise equipment. But balance exercise with rest.

Talk to your doctor before starting to exercise. They know your health best and can tell you what exercise is good and safe for you. Begin with easy exercises like walking or stretching. As you get stronger, you can do more. It's okay if you can't exercise some days—the goal is to help your body, not push it too hard.

Not smoking

Smoking can make pancreatic cancer worse, and quitting can help your body in many ways. If you're a smoker, it's never too late to quit. There are many resources available to help you stop smoking.

Avoid Dehydration

You might find it hard to drink enough when you're sick, especially when you're getting chemotherapy. Having a fever or sweating a lot can also make you dehydrated, which means your body doesn't have enough water. This can happen in just a few hours. Severe dehydration can throw off the normal balance of chemicals in your body. A little thirst is usually okay but being truly dehydrated can be bad for your health. The Mayo Clinic says the following things about dehydration:

> Dehydration can lead to serious complications, including:
>
> - **Heat injury:** If you do not drink enough fluids when you're exercising vigorously and perspiring heavily, you may end up with a heat injury, ranging in severity from mild heat cramps to heat exhaustion or potentially life-threatening heatstroke.
>
> - **Urinary and kidney problems:** Prolonged or repeated bouts of dehydration can cause urinary tract infections, kidney stones, and even kidney failure.
>
> - **Seizures:** Electrolytes—such as potassium and sodium—help carry electrical signals from cell to cell. If your electrolytes are out of balance, the normal electrical messages can become mixed up, which can lead to involuntary muscle contractions and sometimes to a loss of consciousness.
>
> - **Low blood volume shock (hypovolemic shock):** This is one of the most serious, and sometimes life-threatening, complications of dehydration. It occurs when low blood volume causes a drop in blood pressure and a drop in the amount of oxygen in your body.[191]

---

191. Mayo Foundation for Medical Education and Research. (2021, October 14). Dehydration. *Mayo Clinic*. Retrieved from https://www.mayoclinic.org/diseases-conditions/dehydration/symptoms-causes/syc-20354086

To avoid getting dehydrated, you can drink more than just water. You can also have gelatin, milkshakes, and sports drinks (make sure they don't have too much caffeine).

Drinking too much caffeine can dehydrate you. A regular cup of coffee usually has about 100 milligrams of caffeine. Sports drinks, and especially energy drinks, can contain much higher amounts of caffeine, sometimes as much as 500 milligrams, which is considered excessive. Always check the labels to see how much caffeine is in what you're drinking. If you're not sure how much caffeine is okay for you, it's a good idea to talk to your doctor or a dietitian.

You should tell your doctor if you get so dehydrated that you feel dizzy when you stand up. If your dehydration gets bad, you might need to get fluids through an IV, which is a tube that goes into your vein. You can get this at home or at a medical facility. IV fluid can fix your dehydration but won't stop it from happening again.

Supplements

AI helped me write about taking vitamins, micronutrients, and other supplements if you have pancreatic cancer. First, let's learn what these things are. Vitamins and micronutrients are small things that our bodies need to work right, like vitamin C, which helps our immune system. Supplements are like extra food we can take to ensure we're getting enough of these things. But sometimes, they can act like a drug, or as powerfully as a drug, in your body, so it's important to talk to your doctor about them. The FDA says there are about 29,000 supplements you can buy.[192]

Let's discuss the good and bad points about taking supplements and what you might want to ask your cancer doctor about:

Pros:

- **Boosting the immune system:** Vitamins and supplements like vitamin C and Zinc might help strengthen your immune system, which is very important when fighting cancer.

- **Help with side effects:** Sometimes, cancer treatments can make you feel sick, and certain supplements may help with these side effects. For example, ginger can help with nausea, a common side effect of chemotherapy.

- **Improve energy and wellbeing:** When you're sick, losing your appetite and not eating as much happens easily. This can make you feel weak and tired. Some supplements can help you feel stronger and more energetic.

---

192. Institute of Medicine (US) and National Research Council (US) Committee on the Framework for Evaluating the Safety of Dietary Supplements. (2005). *Dietary supplements: A framework for evaluating safety*. National Academies Press. Available from https://www.ncbi.nlm.nih.gov/books/NBK216048/

Cons:

- **Interference with treatment:** This one's important. Certain supplements may interfere with the effectiveness of your cancer treatment. For example, vitamins A, C, and E, which are called antioxidants, might not work well with treatments like chemotherapy and radiation, especially if you take them in large amounts.

- **Not enough evidence:** Even though people say many good things about supplements, there's not always enough scientific proof that they help.

- **Possible side effects:** Just like medicines, supplements can also have side effects. Taking too many supplements or consuming too high a dose of a single supplement can be dangerous and may lead to feeling sick.

Discussion with Oncologist

When you talk to your oncologist, be open and honest about what you're considering. Here are some points you might discuss:

- **Safety first:** Ask your doctor if the supplements you're thinking about are safe to use with your treatment plan. The safety of the patient is always the priority.

- **Evidence:** Ask if there's strong evidence that the supplement will help you. Remember, not everything you read online is true.

- **Side effects:** Discuss potential side effects of the supplements. It's important to weigh the benefits against any possible negative effects.

- **Dosage and timing:** If your oncologist approves your use of certain supplements, talk about the correct dosage and timing. You need to make sure you're taking them the right way.

Make sure to talk to your doctor before taking any new medicine or vitamin. Even a seemingly harmless multivitamin can be bad for you if you have pancreatic cancer. Your doctor should know what's good for you and can help you decide what to do.[193]

Usually, taking vitamins or other extra supplements is not a good idea unless a lab test shows you really need them. Our bodies are complicated. Do not make yours your personal chemistry experiment!

I can't cover all the supplements, but let's take a closer look at a few important ones:

- **Vitamin C**

If you have pancreatic cancer and are thinking about taking vitamin C, you should talk to your cancer doctor first. This is really important if you want to take much of

---

193. OpenAI. (2023). ChatGPT [Computer software]. Retrieved from https://www.openai.com/

it into your veins (intravenous/IV). While vitamin C might help reduce some bad side effects,[194] it could also make chemotherapy less effective.[195] Some research says vitamin C can help treat pancreatic cancer,[196] but always ask your doctor first.

Receiving a high dose of vitamin C through IV infusion is not a decision to take lightly. High-dose IV vitamin C means you're getting much more than the usual daily amount you'd take by mouth. In medical settings, high doses can be from about 10 grams (which is 10,000 milligrams) all the way up to 100 grams (or 100,000 milligrams) for each treatment. At these high levels, vitamin C is more like a medicine than just a regular vitamin, and it's really important that doctors are in charge of this kind of treatment.

- **Iron supplements**

    People with stomach cancers, including pancreatic cancer, might not have enough iron for three reasons: not eating

---

194. Carr, A. C., Vissers, M. C., & Cook, J. S. (2014, October 16). The effect of intravenous vitamin C on cancer- and chemotherapy-related fatigue and quality of life. *Frontiers in Oncology, 4*, Article 283. https://doi.org/10.3389/fonc.2014.00283
195. Heaney, M. L., Gardner, J. R., Karasavvas, N., Golde, D. W., Scheinberg, D. A., Smith, E. A., & O'Connor, O. A. (2008, October 1). Vitamin C antagonizes the cytotoxic effects of antineoplastic drugs. *Cancer Research, 68*(19), 8031-8038. https://doi.org/10.1158/0008-5472.CAN-08-1490
196. Cieslak, J. A., & Cullen, J. J. (2015). Treatment of pancreatic cancer with pharmacological ascorbate. *Current Pharmaceutical Biotechnology, 16*(9), 759-770. https://doi.org/10.2174/1389201016091507151359215

enough iron-rich foods, their body not properly absorbing the iron, and losing blood.[197] It's a good idea to get checked for low iron.[198]

If you don't have enough iron, your doctor might tell you to take iron pills. These pills can help you feel less tired and improve your day-to-day life. But remember, people with pancreatic cancer might feel tired for many reasons, so even if you take iron pills, you might still feel a bit tired.[199]

- **Paricalcitol**

    Here is another supplement to ask your doctor about. There's a special kind of vitamin D called paricalcitol. It's unique because it can interfere with how pancreatic cancer cells shield themselves from our body's defenses.[200] This is good because it's harder for the cancer cells to hide from our immune system. However, the regular vitamin D you find in stores is different and won't do this job. So,

---

197. Verraes, K., & Prenen, H. (2015). Iron deficiency in gastrointestinal oncology. *Annals of Gastroenterology, 28*(1), 19-24.
198. Heaney, M. L., Gardner, J. R., Karasavvas, N., Golde, D. W., Scheinberg, D. A., Smith, E. A., & O'Connor, O. A. (2008). Vitamin C antagonizes the cytotoxic effects of antineoplastic drugs. *Cancer Research, 68*(19), 8031-8038. https://doi.org/10.1158/0008-5472.can-08-1490
199. Verraes, K., & Prenen, H. (2015). Iron deficiency in gastrointestinal oncology. *Annals of Gastroenterology, 28*(1), 19-24. https://www.ncbi.nlm.nih.gov/pmc/articles/PMC4289999/
200. Salk Institute for Biological Studies. (2014, September 25). Modified vitamin D shows promise as treatment for pancreatic cancer. http://www.salk.edu/news-release/modified-vitamin-d-shows-promise-as-treatment-for-pancreatic-cancer/

you shouldn't replace paricalcitol with regular vitamin D supplements.

- **Resveratrol**

Resveratrol is a substance found in red grape skin. Some research suggests it might help treat pancreatic cancer,[201, 202] but it's not proven and it's not a cure. Resveratrol can also have side effects. It can make someone bleed more easily[203] and affect some tumors in a way similar to estrogen, increasing the growth of cancer cells that have estrogen receptors.[204]

---

201. Qin, T., Cheng, L., Xiao, Y., Qian, W., Li, J., Wu, Z., Wang, Z., Xu, Q., Duan, W., Wong, L., Wu, E., Ma, Q., & Ma, J. (2020). NAF-1 inhibition by resveratrol suppresses cancer stem cell-like properties and the invasion of pancreatic cancer. *Frontiers in Oncology, 10*, 1038. https://doi.org/10.3389/fonc.2020.01038

202. Vendrely, V., Peuchant, E., Buscail, E., Moranvillier, I., Rousseau, B., Bedel, A., Brillac, A., de Verneuil, H., Moreau-Gaudry, F., & Dabernat, S. (2017). Resveratrol and capsaicin used together as food complements reduce tumor growth and rescue full efficiency of low dose gemcitabine in a pancreatic cancer model. *Cancer Letters, 390*, 91-102. https://doi.org/10.1016/j.canlet.2017.01.002

203. WebMD. (2022, November 23). Resveratrol: Health benefits, safety information, dosage, and more. Retrieved from https://www.webmd.com/diet/health-benefits-resveratrol

204. Gehm, B. D., McAndrews, J. M., Chien, P. Y., & Jameson, J. L. (1997, December 9). Resveratrol, a polyphenolic compound found in grapes and wine, is an agonist for the estrogen receptor. *Proceedings of the National Academy of Sciences of the United States of America, 94*(25), 14138-14143. https://doi.org/10.1073/pnas.94.25.14138

Family Risk

Unfortunately, Maria Menounos is the latest celebrity to have pancreatic cancer. This is part of her interview on *Today*:

Hoda Kotb:
Longtime entertainment journalist, Maria Menounos, is opening up about her health battle.

Craig Melvin:
And now for the first time she's revealing her stage two pancreatic cancer diagnosis.

Al Roker:
But the great news is Maria says God granted her a miracle. Not only is she cancer free, but she's also expecting her first baby... a cautionary tale because we hear so many times how doctors sometimes dismiss, especially, what women are saying.

Maria Menounos:
Thanks. It's so good to see you... I kept feeling this throbbing in my upper left... lot of people are asking questions, "How did she know? What are the early signs?" ... The TMI [Too Much Information] is loose stool. I had diarrhea for a month and a half. I did all the stool tests. Nothing came back [all tests results were normal].

I was having this throbbing and I kept telling people, "This doesn't feel right." Then I had bouts of severe abdominal pain and then it would go away... normally, I would be like, "Okay, cool, it's over with. Get back to work." I kept trying to get to the bottom of it.

So, the other message is, if the pain persists and your doctors don't know what's going on, go to an outside facility like this and get an outside MRI [such as Prenuvo[205]] because they're incentivized to find something. I know they're not covered by insurance.[206]

In People magazine,[207] Maria said that one of her first symptoms was excruciating pain on a flight after eating a farro salad. Of course, she could not imagine she had pancreatic cancer from her early symptoms.

By the time one has symptoms, pancreatic cancer has usually spread. However, not in every case; Maria "...had a stage 2 pancreatic neuroendocrine tumor, meaning it was contained within the pancreas. Thankfully, it was caught early enough to remove the tumor and cancer cells via surgery without chemotherapy."[208]

---

205. Prenuvo. (n.d.). Retrieved from https://www.prenuvo.com/
206. YouTube. (2023). Maria Menounos on missed symptoms of pancreatic cancer [Video]. YouTube. Retrieved July 15, 2023, from https://youtu.be/xjOVbCjkd9o
207. Etienne, V. (2023, November 1). Maria Menounos felt like she was going to "explode inside" due to "severe" pain from pancreatic cancer. *Peoplemag*. https://people.com/maria-menounos-felt-like-explode-inside-due-to-pancreatic-cancer-8385611
208. Blanton, K. (2023, July 13). Maria Menounos shows off surgery scars in bikini selfie, fans flood her with support. *Prevention*. https://www.prevention.com/health/a44517724/maria-menounos-pancreatic-cancer-surgery-scars-bikini-fans-react-instagram-photo/

Genetics

If someone has pancreatic cancer, it's important that they get genetic testing. This test can be done by drawing some blood or swabbing the inside of their mouth. They should also talk with a professional who knows a lot about genes and family history, a genetic counselor. It's also very important to look closely at their blood relatives' health histories and causes of death.[209]

A little over 10% of pancreatic cancers are from having bad genes.[210, 211] Several are known and can be identified with laboratory testing:

- **TP53**—Li-Fraumini Syndrome[212]

---

209. DeMarco, C. (2022, February 10). Is pancreatic cancer hereditary? 9 things to know. *MD Anderson Cancer Center.* https://www.mdanderson.org/cancerwise/is-pancreatic-cancer-hereditary--9-things-to-know.h00-159537378.html
210. Grover, S., & Syngal, S. (2010, October). Hereditary pancreatic cancer. *Gastroenterology.* https://www.ncbi.nlm.nih.gov/pmc/articles/PMC3149791/
211. PanCAN. (2021, November 17). Genetics and hereditary factors of pancreatic cancer. *Pancreatic Cancer Action Network.* Retrieved from https://pancan.org/facing-pancreatic-cancer/about-pancreatic-cancer/risk-factors/genetic-hereditary/
212. Aversa, J. G., De Abreu, F. B., Yano, S., Xi, L., Hadley, D. W., Manoli, I., Raffeld, M., Sadowski, S. M., & Nilubol, N. (2020, March 30). The first pancreatic neuroendocrine tumor in Li-Fraumeni syndrome: A case report. *BMC Cancer, 20*(1), 256. https://doi.org/10.1186/s12885-020-06723-6

Living with Pancreatic Cancer: A Patient and Family Guide

- **P16**[213, 214]

- **PALB2**[215]

- **BRCA 1** and **BRCA 2**

- **CDKN2A**

- **PRSS1**—familial pancreatitis

- **STK11**—Peutz-Jeghers Syndrome

- **VHL**—Von Hippel-Lindau Syndrome

- **NF1 and MEN1**—Pancreatic neuroendocrine tumors (PNETs)[216]

---

213. Iwatate, Y., Hoshino, I., Ishige, F., Itami, M., Chiba, S., Arimitsu, H., Yanagibashi, H., Nagase, H., Yokota, H., & Takayama, W. (2020, July). Prognostic significance of p16 protein in pancreatic ductal adenocarcinoma. *Molecular and Clinical Oncology, 13*(1), 83-91. https://doi.org/10.3892/mco.2020.2047

214. Jeong, J., Park, Y. N., Park, J. S., Yoon, D. S., Chi, H. S., & Kim, B. R. (2005, August 31). Clinical significance of p16 protein expression loss and aberrant p53 protein expression in pancreatic cancer. *Yonsei Medical Journal, 46*(4), 519-525. https://doi.org/10.3349/ymj.2005.46.4.519

215. Hofstatter, E. W., Domchek, S. M., Miron, A., Garber, J., Wang, M., Componeschi, K., Boghossian, L., Miron, P. L., Nathanson, K. L., & Tung, N. (2011, June). PALB2 mutations in familial breast and pancreatic cancer. *Familial Cancer, 10*(2), 225-231. https://doi.org/10.1007/s10689-011-9426-1

216. Kuhlmann, C. (2018, October 8). Inherited gene mutations and pancreatic cancer. *Seena Magowitz Foundation*. Retrieved from https://seenamagowitzfoundation.org/six-inherited-genetic-mutations-likned-to-increased-risk-of-pancreatic-cancer/

"Only about 7% will have an inheritable germline mutation, such as BRCA, detected in testing. Another 5% or so will have a family history of pancreatic cancer, not a known mutation."[217] The reason might be that several different genes, which are not perfect or have some issues, are working together to cause the cancer. That's called "polygenic." There could be undiscovered genes that cause or make it more likely to get pancreatic cancer. Also, a person can get pancreatic cancer by chance, not because it's inherited, even if it tends to occur in their family.

If you or a family member learns you carry a gene that increases the risk for pancreatic cancer, it's smart for your immediate family—like parents, siblings, and children—to also get tested.

If a family member finds out they have genes that might make them more likely to get pancreatic cancer, they should talk to their regular doctor about it. This is important because these genes can also make them more likely to get other types of cancer and illnesses.

If someone in your family has a gene that might make them more likely to get pancreatic cancer, it's also a good idea to talk to a genetic counselor. Per AI, here's what a genetic counselor can do:

---

217. DeMarco, C. (2022, February 10). Is pancreatic cancer hereditary? 9 things to know. *MD Anderson Cancer Center*. https://www.mdanderson.org/cancerwise/is-pancreatic-cancer-hereditary--9-things-to-know.h00-159537378.html

- **Figure out the risk:** They'll look at your family history and might ask for a special test to see if you have a gene that could increase your risk for pancreatic cancer.

- **Explain the test results:** If you do have a risk gene, they'll explain what that means. Just because you have the gene doesn't mean you'll definitely get cancer. It just means you have a higher chance.

- **Talk about how to stay healthy:** They'll give advice on what you can do to lower your chances of getting cancer. This could be things like regular check-ups, changing your diet, or even certain medications or surgeries.

- **Help with your feelings:** Finding out you have a risk gene can be scary. The counselor can help you handle these feelings.

- **Talk about family:** If you have a risk gene, your family might have it, too. The counselor can help you understand what this means for them.

- **Discuss rules and rights:** They'll talk about how results from genetic testing information can affect things like insurance and jobs. There are laws to protect you, but some things aren't covered like long-term care insurance.

Remember, the job of a genetic counselor is to help you understand complex information about genes and make choices about your health.[218]

The best thing someone can do if they have a higher chance of getting pancreatic cancer because of their genes is to make healthier choices. Most pancreatic cancers are linked to these things we can control:

- **Chronic pancreatitis:** Long-term pancreatic inflammation often develops in people who smoke and use excessive amounts of alcohol.[219]

- **Smoking:** Smoking contributes to the development of pancreatic cancer.

- **Excess weight:** Obesity increases your risk of developing pancreatic cancer.

- **Unhealthy diet:** Eating a lot of red and processed meats and few vegetables puts you at greater risk.[220]

- **Alcohol Consumption:** Heavy alcohol use may increase the risk of pancreatic cancer, particularly in individuals with chronic pancreatitis.

---

218. OpenAI. (2023). ChatGPT [Computer software]. Retrieved from https://www.openai.com/
219. Lavarone, K. (2023). What is the link between alcohol and pancreatic cancer? *Medical News Today.* https://www.medicalnewstoday.com/articles/what-causes-pancreatic-cancer-alcohol
220. Pennmedicine.org. (2023). Pancreatic cancer risks and prevention. Retrieved from https://www.pennmedicine.org/cancer/types-of-cancer/pancreatic-cancer/pancreatic-cancer-risks-and-prevention

- **Physical Inactivity:** A sedentary lifestyle may increase the risk, whereas regular physical activity is beneficial.

- **Diabetes:** Long-standing diabetes is associated with an increased risk of pancreatic cancer.

Testing for Pancreatic Cancer

It's normal for you to worry about other family members possibly having pancreatic cancer or for them to be scared about it, too. Let's break this down into four groups.

I'm putting these topics into groups with particular attention to whether a family member had these signs **before** or **after** they found out you were sick. "Medical Student Syndrome" is when someone, often a medical student or someone who knows a bit about health, starts to think they have the symptoms of an illness after learning about it. If this worry comes from reading online, it's called "cyberchondria."

Here are some things you might notice if you have pancreatic cancer:

- Pain in your stomach that you may also feel in your back

- Not feeling hungry or losing weight without trying

- Skin and eyes turning yellow (this is called jaundice)

- Poop that is light-colored and/or floats

- Pee that is dark-colored

- Skin that itches a lot

- Being told you have diabetes, or if you already have diabetes, it's getting harder to control.

- Blood clots

- Feeling really tired all the time.

- Unintentional weight loss[221]

- Diarrhea

Group 1—Very Uncommon:

Situation: If someone in your family, like a mom, dad, sibling, or adult child, finds out they have a risk gene that makes it more likely to get pancreatic cancer, and they have symptoms **before** they knew about your pancreatic cancer.

Recommendation: In that case, they should see a stomach doctor (a gastroenterologist). They might need special tests like an

---

221. Johns Hopkins Medicine. (2021, August 8). Pancreatic cancer symptoms. Retrieved from https://www.hopkinsmedicine.org/health/conditions-and-diseases/pancreatic-cancer/pancreatic-cancer-symptoms

MRI, or a camera test called an endoscopic ultrasound (EUS) to check for pancreatic cancer.[222]

Group 2—Uncommon:

Situation: If you have a blood relative who tested positive for a gene that increases the risk of pancreatic cancer but did not experience these symptoms until **after** they were aware of your condition.

Recommendation: They should consult a specialized GI doctor (gastroenterologist) who focuses on pancreatic cancer. Regular tests conducted by a health care professional with expertise in early detection of pancreatic cancer are necessary. However, statistically, the odds are strongly in their favor of not developing the disease. Be aware of "cyberchondria," especially if these worries increase after reading about the condition online. Symptoms like pain, fatigue, and weight loss can sometimes be more related to stress or worry than cancer.

Group 3—Pretty Common:

Situation: The symptoms listed above also happen to many people who don't have a special gene that makes them more likely to get pancreatic cancer. Usually, these symptoms are easy to treat and aren't because of pancreatic cancer.

---

222. American Cancer Society. (2019, February 11). Can pancreatic cancer be found early? Retrieved from https://www.cancer.org/cancer/types/pancreatic-cancer/detection-diagnosis-staging/detection.html

Recommendation: The tests to find out if they do or don't have pancreatic cancer can be expensive and time-consuming. If they have insurance other than Medicare, prior authorization may be needed for some tests. Anyone in this group should see a GI doctor to determine if testing for pancreatic cancer is necessary. An MRI, costing about $500 out-of-pocket, is an option and doesn't use radiation.

Group 4—Most Common Group:

Situation: People in this group don't have genes that make them more likely to get cancer and don't show any symptoms either. However, they might still worry if they have a close relative with pancreatic cancer.

Recommendation: Pancreatic cancer is relatively rare, and the level of worry will often exceed the risk. While not routinely recommended, additional testing could be considered. Options include a liquid biopsy, a new type of blood test, or opting for an annual MRI. An MRI, which does not use radiation, is slightly more effective than a CT scan in detecting pancreatic cancer. According to MD Anderson Cancer Center, there is no standard screening test for healthy adults for pancreatic cancer. Dr. Maitra from the center cautions that screening everyone over age 50 could lead to a large number of false positives, unnecessary anxiety, and needless tests without meaningful outcomes.[223]

---

223. Underferth, D. (2019a, November 6). Can you screen for pancreatic cancer? *MD Anderson Cancer Center.* Retrieved from https://www.mdanderson.org/publications/focused-on-health/can-you-screen-for-pancreatic-cancer-.h20-1592991.html

Considerations: Not everyone in Group 4 requires the same approach. Their level of concern and overall health are key factors in determining the next steps. Hopefully, in the near future, doctors might be able to better judge both general and specific risks for pancreatic cancer using AI technology. They could also advise patients on ways to lower their risk and recommend appropriate screening tests.[224]

Screening for Pancreatic Cancer:

While the rest of this book is for patients, these two paragraphs are for policymakers. I have an idea for detecting pancreatic cancer without requiring additional scans. This idea is inspired by studies from Massachusetts General Hospital and the Massachusetts Institute of Technology, which demonstrated that AI can outperform doctors in identifying breast cancer in mammograms.[225] Similarly, we could apply AI to detect pancreatic cancer early by analyzing standard scans that patients already receive, such as CTs, MRIs, and ultrasounds. Even if these scans were not specifically targeting the pancreas, given the difficulty in detecting pancreatic cancer, we might discover it incidentally. For instance, when scanning for gallbladder issues, the pancreas is also imaged, providing an opportunity to identify cancer early.

---

224. OpenAI. (2023). ChatGPT [Computer software]. Retrieved from https://www.openai.com/
225. Yala, A., et al. (2021). Toward robust mammography-based models for breast cancer risk. *Science Translational Medicine, 13*(589), eaba4373. https://doi.org/10.1126/scitranslmed.aba4373

For this approach to work, AI needs to study a dataset that contains thousands of images of pancreases, both with and without cancer. This training will enable it to discern the differences and assist doctors in identifying cancer sooner. The challenge lies in convincing radiologists to trust and adopt this AI tool. Integrating the AI screening tool directly into the imaging machines could automate the process. Moreover, helping doctors understand the AI's findings by highlighting the specific areas in the images indicative of cancer could foster trust in this technology.

As briefly mentioned in the Hope chapter, the FDA has approved a new test. The test is called Galleri, created by a company named Grail. This test is special because it can find pancreatic cancer and other cancers using a simple blood test.[226]

The Galleri test looks for very small amounts of pancreatic tumor DNA, like the cancer's blueprint, in your blood. It's pretty good at finding pancreatic cancer, with a success rate of 84%. That means it can correctly find cancer 84 out of 100 times.[227] It's not perfect, but it's pretty good.

But there's a downside—the test is pretty expensive. It costs about $1,000 ($$$ According to our grouping). And the

---

226. Tirumalaraju, D. (2019, May 15). Grail gets FDA breakthrough designation for multi-cancer test. *Medical Device Network*. https://www.medicaldevice-network.com/news/grail-test-fda-breakthrough-status/

227. Galleri® Test. (2023). Test performance: Deeper dive for health care providers. Retrieved from https://www.galleri.com/hcp/galleri-test-performance

company recommends you take this test every year. The cost would really add up over time.

Back in 2012, a 15-year-old award-winning student named Jack Andraka, made news by creating a low-cost test to detect pancreatic cancer early. A 2020 article from GI Alliance noted, "Andraka's test is in the patent process and will not be available to markets for years"[228] but didn't explain why it's taking so long to become available to the public.

Jack's test is based on his discovery that a protein, mesothelin, is overproduced by pancreatic cancers.[229, 230] Blood samples from those with pancreatic cancer have more mesothelin than normal people. As a result of Jack's work, there is research on using mesothelin overproduction as a basis for drugs and vaccines.[231]

The Swedish company, Immunova, is hoping to offer an early detection test for pancreatic cancer in 2024. For a short

---

228. GI Alliance. (2020, February 14). New pancreatic cancer test developed by 15-year-old, Jack Andraka. *GI Alliance: Nation's Premier Gastroenterology Practice.* https://gialliance.com/gastroenterology-blog/new-pancreatic-cancer-test-developed-by-15-year-old-jack-andraka

229. Tucker, A. (2012, December 1). Jack Andraka, the teen prodigy of pancreatic cancer. *Smithsonian.com.* https://www.smithsonianmag.com/science-nature/jack-andraka-the-teen-prodigy-of-pancreatic-cancer-135925809

230. GI Alliance. (2020, February 14). New pancreatic cancer test developed by 15-year-old, Jack Andraka. *GI Alliance: Nation's Premier Gastroenterology Practice.* https://gialliance.com/gastroenterology-blog/new-pancreatic-cancer-test-developed-by-15-year-old-jack-andraka

231. Lv, J., & Li, P. (2019). Mesothelin as a biomarker for targeted therapy. *Biomarker Research, 7*(1). https://doi.org/10.1186/s40364-019-0169-8

time, they had a test, IMMray PanCan-d, on the market for detecting pancreatic cancer but it was withdrawn because it did not perform up to expectations.[232]

---

232. Immunovia. (2023, July 11). Immunovia to significantly restructure to focus resources on its next-generation blood test for pancreatic cancer detection—IMMUNOVIA—investor relations. Retrieved from https://investor.immunovia.com/immunovia-to-significantly-restructure-to-focus-resources-on-its-next-generation-blood-test-for-pancreatic-cancer-detection/

Financial Aspects

There were financial fears (both my husband and I missing work) as we moved to Houston. Again, God was very generous to us. Every time we turned around, someone unknown to us was being kind and generous. It allowed me not to worry so much about the financial aspects of our situation and concentrate more on just getting well. **KH**

Everyone should be able to get the best cancer treatments, no matter how much money they have. If you have little money, you may need to do some extra things to get good care. For example, you could look for charities or research studies to help you. This can take time, but it's worth it. This book tells you about groups that want to help you. Jules Johnston and I also give you ideas on how to raise money for your medical bills.

Understanding and Dealing with Health Insurance (AI assisted)

When you're dealing with pancreatic cancer, it's important to know about health insurance. Different people have different types of insurance, meaning you might have to pay extra money sometimes, like deductibles and co-pays.

Your health insurance doesn't say it will give you the best medical treatment. It just promises to do what the papers you signed say it will do. This means only certain treatments for pancreatic cancer might be paid for by your insurance. To know what's covered, you should look at your insurance papers. These papers could have names like "Summary of Benefits and Coverage," "Benefit Language," or "Evidence of Coverage." It's important to know what your insurance pays for.

Health insurance plans must follow privacy laws, like the Health Insurance Portability and Accountability Act (HIPAA) in the United States. These laws make sure your medical information stays private and isn't shared without your permission.

So, while the company's leaders may choose the type of plan they offer to employees, they can't look at your personal medical records or change your benefits based on your specific health needs. If you have questions about what your plan covers, it's best to talk to the insurance company directly or check your benefits guide.[233]

Early health insurance was much different:

A group of schoolteachers in Dallas who joined forces with Baylor University Hospital to "prepay" for their health

---

233. OpenAI. (2023). ChatGPT [Computer software]. Retrieved from https://www.openai.com/

care at a premium of 50 cents per person, per month. This model is largely referenced as the first modern commercial hospital insurance plan, and evolved directly into an organization you may have heard of called Blue Cross. In return for paying 50 cents per teacher, per month, school systems were guaranteed their teachers could spend up to 21 days in the hospital at no cost.[234]

Those lucky enough to be healthy provided their funds to care for the sick. This was called risk pooling. While it is a term still used, the meaning of risk pooling has evolved away from insurers being passive payers.

Insurance companies aren't just sitting back and paying out money anymore. They're taking a more active role, like making deals to lower the cost of medicine or giving people incentives to stay healthy. So, while we still use the term "risk pooling," it's important to remember that its meaning has changed.

Today, health insurers play a direct role in cancer care through selective payment. Preauthorization, which is also known as precertification or prior approval, has become a very important concept. Except in an emergency, before your health insurance will pay for costly tests, treatments or procedures, your doctor and insurance company have to agree it's necessary. Preauthorization means getting permission before medical treatment or testing is done. This includes knowing which

---

234. Lichtenstein, E. (2023, July 10). The history of health insurance: Past, present, and future. *AgentSync*. https://agentsync.io/blog/loa/the-history-of-health-insurance-past-present-and-future

treatments your health plan covers, where you can get this care, and who can give it to you. Preauthorization takes a lot of time.

Your doctor usually initiates preauthorization for specialty care like pancreatic cancer treatment. This means the doctor's office will typically contact the insurance company for you. However, it's a good idea for patients to also be involved in this process. You can double-check with your insurance company to make sure that the preauthorization has been approved. This helps you avoid unexpected costs later on.

So, while your doctor's office usually handles the paperwork, being proactive and staying in the loop can help ensure everything goes as smoothly as possible. Always make sure you understand what your insurance covers and what you may be responsible for paying.

> From AI: It is fairly common for initial claims to be denied for various reasons—some accidental, such as clerical errors, and others more systematic, like the treatment being out-of-network or deemed not medically necessary. Appealing these decisions can sometimes lead to a reversal, depending on the specifics of the case and the insurance policy's guidelines.
>
> Many health insurance plans have tiered appeal processes that may involve multiple levels of review, including an internal review by the insurance company and an external review by an independent third party. The probability of an appeal being successful can depend on many factors,

including the quality of the medical evidence presented and the specifics of the insurance policy.

If you're frequently denied coverage initially but are approved upon appeal, consult with a patient advocate or legal advisor familiar with your jurisdiction's health insurance laws and regulations. Such professionals can offer advice tailored to your specific situation and help you navigate the appeals process more effectively.[235]

There have been problems with the preauthorization system in the past.

Before health insurers reject claims for medical reasons, company doctors must review them, according to insurance laws and regulations in many states. Medical directors are expected to examine patient records, review coverage policies and use their expertise to decide whether to approve or deny claims, regulators said. This process helps avoid unfair denials.

But the Cigna review system that blocked van Terheyden's claim bypasses those steps. Medical directors do not see any patient records or put their medical judgment to use, said former company employees familiar with the system. Instead, a computer does the work. A Cigna algorithm flags mismatches between diagnoses and what the company considers acceptable tests and procedures for those

---

235. OpenAI. (2023). ChatGPT [Computer software]. Retrieved from https://www.openai.com/

ailments. Company doctors then sign off on the denials in batches, according to interviews with former employees who spoke on condition of anonymity.

"We literally click and submit," one former Cigna doctor said. "It takes all of 10 seconds to do 50 at a time."[236]

The quote above is about lab tests. It is an example of that some insurance companies can be too quick in saying "no" to covering medical costs. This can happen for a lot of reasons. Maybe a hospital has a special way of treating pancreatic cancer that's different and better. Your insurance company might not agree. They might not cover the costs.

When a traditional doctor's office has to fight with the insurance company to get a claim approved, it takes up a lot of time. This is a big job for the people who work there. On the other hand, a concierge doctor ($$$) has fewer patients. This means they can spend more time making sure all the paperwork is correct. They even wait on the phone for a long time to talk directly with the insurance company's doctor. This can make a big difference in getting things approved.

A different type of health insurance is a Health Maintenance Organization (HMO). It is a type of health insurance with strict rules about where to go for cancer treatment. It usually wants you to see doctors and go to hospitals that are part of its own network.

---

236. Rucker, P., Miller, M., & Armstrong, D. (2023, March 25). How Cigna saves millions by having its doctors reject claims without reading them. *ProPublica.* https://www.propublica.org/article/cigna-pxdx-medical-health-insurance-rejection-claims

So, if you want to go to a really good and famous place for cancer care that's far away, your HMO will not pay for it.

However, some HMOs allow you to get an opinion from an expert outside their network. To know for sure, you should read the Summary of Benefits and Coverage (SB&C) part of your health insurance papers. Make sure to look closely at the sections that talk about what is not covered or has limits.

Another kind of health insurance is called a Preferred Provider Organization, or PPO for short. This plan will help pay for medical services even if they're from doctors or hospitals that aren't on their approved list. But there's a catch: the amount of money the plan covers for these services can be a little or even a lot less than what it covers for approved services.

When your insurance pays less, you have to pay more. This can mean bigger copayments (the fixed amount you pay for a health care service) and larger deductibles (the amount you pay before your insurance starts to pay).

Some jobs offer health insurance that they fund and set up themselves instead of buying health insurance. In this case, the company hires an insurance company to administer the plan, so the company does not know about their employees' medical care.

If your company has this type of plan and your insurance does not cover something, but you think it should, you can talk to your bosses. If you're in a union, they can also help you make your case. Just remember, by doing this, you're letting your company know about any medical issues you have that they are not allowed to know about otherwise.

There used to be a limit or overall maximum that a health insurance company would pay for your health care. It was known by several names such as insurance limit, maximum amount of insurance, and limit of liability. The Affordable Care Act (ACA), which became law in 2010 outlawed this limit. According to the U.S. Department of Health and Human Services, "The healthcare law stops insurance companies from limiting yearly or lifetime coverage expenses for essential health benefits."[237] Pancreatic cancer health care certainly falls under the category of essential health benefits.

Doctors usually treat pancreatic cancer with treatments that are standard and covered by insurance, which often go hand in hand. However, there can be new, promising, and expensive treatments insurance won't cover. We have to face the fact that how much money you have can impact your medical treatment.

If you have insurance, you might be able to get them to cover tests and treatments that they don't usually pay for. But the key to getting this money is understanding how your insurance works. You can ask for help from the Patient Advocate Foundation,[238] which provides resources on these topics.

---

237. U.S. Department of Health and Human Services. (2023, August 31). Lifetime & annual limits. Retrieved from https://www.hhs.gov/healthcare/about-the-aca/benefit-limits/

238. Patient Advocate Foundation. (n.d.). Retrieved from https://www.patientadvocate.org/

Insurance companies usually have information on their websites about how to get treatments approved. But this info is often difficult to understand. It's good to call the company's help center to learn more. Hopefully, the person you talk to will give you helpful advice.

It's important to follow all the rules. If you don't, the insurance company might not pay for your treatment. For example, if you get a treatment without getting the needed preauthorization, you almost certainly will have to pay for it yourself.

If you think about joining a medical study to get a promising new treatment given the thumbs up by FDA, there's some good news! Some insurance companies, even HMOs, are now willing to pay for these studies as long as they happen within their own network.

Some other medical studies get money from research funds or drug companies. Suppose you join these studies and bring a helper like a family member. In that case, you'll usually get paid back for extra costs like travel, staying somewhere, and meals.

When you are eligible for Medicare you will have a choice between traditional Medicare and Medicare Advantage programs. One very big advantage of traditional Medicare is, "Medicare, including Part A, rarely requires prior authorization."[239]

---

239. Esch, J. (2021, September 27). Medicare prior authorization explained. *Medicare FAQ*. Retrieved from https://www.medicarefaq.com/faqs/medicare-prior-authorization/

I rarely, if ever, recommend Medicare Advantage programs to my patients. AI details why:

First, Medicare Advantage is like an "all-in-one" package combining Original Medicare (Part A and Part B) with extra benefits like vision, dental, and sometimes even gym memberships. Sounds great, right? Well, there are some downsides, too:

1. **Limited Network of Doctors:** With Medicare Advantage, you usually have to pick your doctors and hospitals from a list. If your favorite doctor isn't on that list, you might have to pay more to see them.

2. **More Rules:** Sometimes, you need a "referral" to see a specialist. This means you have to get permission from another doctor first. This can take time and be a real hassle.

3. **Cost Can Be Deceptive:** Even though the monthly cost might seem lower, you often have to pay when you get services, like visiting a doctor. These costs can add up quickly.

4. **Change in Benefits:** The benefits you get can change each year. Something that was covered this year might not be covered next year.

5. **Coverage Area:** If you move or travel a lot, your plan might not work well in different places. Some plans only work in certain areas, so if you're someone who likes to move around, this could be a problem.

6. **Complicated to Switch:** It can be complicated if you want to switch back to Original Medicare. You might also have trouble getting a "Medigap" plan, which is extra insurance that works with Original Medicare but not with Medicare Advantage.

7. **Prescription Drug Limitations:** Some Medicare Advantage plans have prescription drug coverage, but the list of covered drugs might be limited. You might pay more for your medication.

So, while Medicare Advantage plans might offer extra perks, they come with some rules and limitations you won't find with Original Medicare. Thinking about what's most important to you before making a choice is essential.[240]

Choosing your Medicare plan isn't always easy. Traditional/normal Medicare is what most older people in the United States use. It does not pay for prescription medicines unless you pay extra for a Medicare Part D plan. It is insurance that helps pay for most (not all) prescription drugs. Almost everyone with pancreatic cancer, should buy a Medicare Part D plan. Let's read what AI says about the good and not-so-good things about Medicare Part D, as well as how much it costs.

---

240. OpenAI. (2023). ChatGPT [Computer software]. Retrieved from https://www.openai.com/

Advantages:

1. **Helps with Medicine Costs:** Medicare Part D helps people afford the medications they need. This is a big deal because medicine can be really expensive.

2. **Choice of Plans:** You can pick from different plans to find one that covers the medications you take.

3. **Wider Access:** With a Part D plan, you're not limited to just one pharmacy. You can go to any pharmacy that accepts Medicare.

4. **Safety Nets:** Some plans offer "catastrophic coverage." This means if you spend a lot on medications, the plan will cover even more of the costs.

Disadvantages:

1. **Complexity:** Picking a plan can be confusing. There are lots of options and details to understand.

2. **Coverage Gap:** There's something called the "donut hole." This is a gap where you have to pay more out of pocket for your medicines, after you've already spent a certain amount.

3. **Not All Drugs Covered:** Some medicines might not be covered by your plan, or you might need special permission for certain drugs.

4. **Additional Cost:** You pay for Part D in addition to other Medicare costs. That means more money out of your pocket.

Cost:

1. **Monthly Premium:** You'll have to pay an extra fee every month for Part D. This fee varies depending on the plan you choose.

2. **Deductible:** This is the amount you pay for medications before the plan starts to help. Deductibles can range from $0 to a few hundred dollars per year.

3. **Copayments and Coinsurance:** Once the deductible is met, you'll still need to pay a small part of the medicine cost, called a copayment or coinsurance.

So, Medicare Part D has its upsides and downsides. It helps with the cost of medications but can be confusing and has some extra costs. Before choosing a plan, it's a good idea to look at all the details and talk to a health care expert to make sure it's the right fit for you.[241]

Some cancer treatments, like getting medicine through a needle in your vein, are part of your medical benefits. This is different from your pharmacy benefits, which cover things like pills. Each type of treatment might have a small fee you need to pay.

---

241. OpenAI. (2023). ChatGPT [Computer software]. Retrieved from https://www.openai.com/

Some chemo comes as pills. Those pills are covered by your pharmacy benefits, not your medical benefits. So, when choosing a health plan like Part D, you need to think carefully. It's a good idea to look at everything and talk to a health care expert to make sure the plan is right for you.

Also, there are special programs called the Medicare Savings Programs.[242] This is for people who have Medicare but don't have a lot of money and can't get Medicaid.

Federal Governmental Support

Family Medical Leave Act (FMLA)

One of the patients, **KH**, who contributed to this book said that using FMLA helped her. The FMLA is a law in the United States that gives workers certain rights if they or their family members get sick. AI lists some of the benefits:

1. **Keeping Your Job:** The main point of FMLA is to make sure you don't lose your job if you have to take some time off for valid family or medical reasons. You can be gone up to 12 weeks in one year and still have your job when you come back.

2. **Reasons for Leave:** You can use FMLA for several reasons, including if taking care of a very sick family member (like your mom, dad, or child) or if you are too sick to work.

---

242. Medicare. (2023). Medicare Savings Programs. Retrieved from https://www.medicare.gov/medicare-savings-programs

3. **Health Insurance:** Even though you're not at work, your employer must keep your health insurance going as if you were still there. This means you won't lose health coverage while on FMLA leave.

4. **Peace of Mind:** Knowing you won't lose your job if you're sick or need to care for a family member can help you feel less stressed.

Remember, FMLA doesn't mean your employer has to pay you while you're not at work. It just says they have to keep your job open for you and continue your health insurance. You might be able to use vacation or sick days, but that depends on your employer's rules.[243]

If you want to use the Family and Medical Leave Act (FMLA) to take time off work, here's what you need to do, per AI:

1. **Check if you can use FMLA:** Make sure you fit the rules for FMLA. You need to have worked for your company for a year, put in at least 1,250 hours of work in the past year, and your workplace must have 50 or more workers within 75 miles.

2. **Tell your boss ahead of time:** You have to tell your boss at least 30 days before you want to start your FMLA time off.

---

243. OpenAI. (2023). ChatGPT [Computer software]. Retrieved from https://www.openai.com/

3. **Fill out the forms:** Your company will give you the FMLA forms you need to fill out. Be sure to fill them out correctly and completely. You should include why you need to take time off and for how long.

4. **Show proof if needed:** Your company will most likely ask for more information, like a doctor's note, to prove why you need to take FMLA time off.

5. **Turn in your FMLA application:** Give your finished forms and any extra information to your company. Remember to keep a copy of everything for yourself.

6. **Wait for your company to decide:** Your boss will take some time to look at your forms and decide if you can take FMLA time off.

7. **Start your FMLA time off:** If your company says yes, follow their instructions to start your time off.

Remember, every company has its own rules and steps for FMLA. To make sure you understand how to apply for FMLA time off at your job, talk to someone in your human resources department or look in your employee handbook.[244]

---

244. OpenAI. (2023). ChatGPT [Computer software]. Retrieved from https://www.openai.com/

Social Security Disability Insurance

Social Security Disability Insurance (SSDI) is a program in the United States that helps people who can't work because of a long-term disability. Per AI, here's what SSDI can provide for those who qualify:

1. **Monthly Money:** The SSDI program gives money each month to those who can't work because of their disability. The amount you get depends on how much money you've earned in the past.

2. **Health Care:** After getting SSDI money for two years, a person can get Medicare. Medicare is a health insurance program that can help pay for doctor visits, hospital stays, and other medical needs, no matter how old the person is.

3. **Family Benefits:** If a person with a disability has children or a spouse who cares for their children, those family members might also be able to receive money from SSDI.

4. **Retirement Money:** If a person is getting SSDI money when they reach the age to retire, they'll start getting retirement money from Social Security.

5. **Help Staying out of Poverty:** SSDI money might not be as much as a person used to earn, but it can still help keep them from being very poor because they can't work.

6. **Support to Go Back to Work:** SSDI has some programs to help people who might be able to return to work. They can keep getting some money while they try to work again, and SSDI might even help pay for training or education.

Remember, not everyone can get SSDI. To qualify, a person has to have worked a certain amount of time and paid into the Social Security system.[245]

You also need to have a disease or other medical condition that qualifies for Compassionate Allowance. Pancreatic cancer qualifies.[246]

Supplemental Security Income (SSI)

If you have pancreatic cancer and live in the United States, you can apply for SSI. You do not need to have paid Social Security taxes to get this income. The Social Security Administration, or SSA, has rules you need to follow. They check medical facts to decide if someone can get benefits. The rules are in a book called the Blue Book. Pancreatic cancer is in Section 13.17, "Malignant Neoplastic Diseases." If you want to learn more, you can look there.

AI adds that to qualify for benefits because of pancreatic cancer, you need to meet some conditions:

---

245. OpenAI. (2023). ChatGPT [Computer software]. Retrieved from https://www.openai.com/
246. Disability Benefits Center. (2023). Compassionate allowance—pancreatic cancer. Retrieved from https://www.disabilitybenefitscenter.org/compassionate-allowances/pancreatic-cancer-social-security-disability

Living with Pancreatic Cancer: A Patient and Family Guide

1. **Diagnosis:** You must have pancreatic cancer, proven by medical records, biopsy results, pathology reports, or imaging studies like CT scans and MRIs.

2. **Severe cancer:** You can usually qualify if your pancreatic cancer is advanced or has spread to other parts of your body.

3. **Inoperable tumor:** The cancer cannot be removed by surgery.

4. **Persistence or recurrence:** You can qualify if the cancer stays or comes back even after treatment or surgery.

5. **Trouble working:** You need to show that the cancer or its treatment makes it hard for you to work. You can prove this with records showing symptoms like pain, tiredness, weight loss, stomach problems, or other issues from the cancer or treatment.

6. **Long-term disability:** The cancer must last at least a year or be life-threatening.

To apply for benefits, fill out the required forms and give them medical records showing pancreatic cancer. This includes documents, reports, scan results, notes about surgery, treatment history, lab reports, and other papers showing how your cancer makes it hard for you to work.[247]

---

247. OpenAI. (2023). ChatGPT [Computer software]. Retrieved from https://www.openai.com/

If you think you can get Social Security Disability Benefits, here's what to do next:

1. **Check if you can apply:** Before you start, make sure you can apply for either Social Security Disability Insurance (SSDI) or Supplemental Security Income (SSI). Again, SSDI is for people who have worked and contributed to Social Security through their jobs. SSI, on the other hand, is for individuals who haven't contributed to Social Security but still need financial assistance.

2. **Talk to your doctors:** Tell your doctors or members of their staff that you want to apply for disability benefits. They can give extra medical advice, check how well you can do everyday tasks, or give additional paperwork to support your case.

3. **Start applying:** There are a few ways to apply for disability benefits. You can apply on the SSA's website (www.ssa.gov), call their free phone number (1-800-772-1213) to set up a meeting or go to your local Social Security office to fill out the application.

4. **Fill out all forms:** Complete the application forms from the SSA. Be clear and give details about your health condition, past jobs, and what you do daily. Make sure to include all important medical records and paperwork as proof.

5. **Think about getting a lawyer:** Even though you don't have to, some people get a lawyer who specializes in Social

Security Disability. They can help guide you through the application process, get proof, and make sure you have a strong case.

6. **Stay in touch and cooperate:** After you send your application, contact the SSA and quickly answer any requests for more information or medical check-ups. Keep copies of all papers and letters related to your case.

7. **Wait for an answer:** The SSA will look over your application and medical proof to decide if you can get benefits. This can take a few months, and you might need to go to a disability hearing if your first application is not accepted.

Remember, this process can change based on your situation and your condition. Because this can be tricky, it might be helpful to talk to a lawyer who specializes in Social Security Disability to make sure you have the best chance of a successful application.[248]

State Government Resources

State-specific resources vary a lot. With the help of AI, here are a few general types of aid you might find:

1. **Medicaid:** This is a state and federal program that provides health coverage for some low-income people, fami-

---

248. OpenAI. (2023). ChatGPT [Computer software]. Retrieved from https://www.openai.com/

lies and children, pregnant women, the elderly, and people with disabilities. If you're eligible, it might cover some costs related to your illness.

2. **State Disability Programs:** Some states offer their own disability benefits programs, separate from the federal SSDI (Social Security Disability Insurance) or SSI (Supplemental Security Income). These may provide financial assistance.

3. **Department of Health Services:** Many states have health departments offering home care, meal delivery, or respite care resources.

4. **Cancer-Specific Programs:** Some states have programs specifically designed for cancer patients. They may offer resources like special insurance programs, medication assistance, transportation to medical appointments, etc.

5. **State-Sponsored Housing Assistance:** For individuals who have become disabled and are not able to work, there may be housing assistance programs available.

6. **Non-Profit Organizations:** While not government-run, numerous non-profit organizations support people with cancer, from emotional support groups to financial aid. Some may be state-specific.

Remember, each state has its own specific programs and eligibility requirements, so it's a good idea to visit your state government's official website or call their Health and Human Services department for the most accurate and current information.[249]

Tapping into Little-Known Funds
(co-written with Guilianna Johnston)

"The [school] district had a shared-leave policy, and I was donated more leave than I could use. I never missed a full paycheck while I was off for almost a year. That alone was a gift." **KH**

Project Purple[250] and The National Pancreas Foundation[251] provide direct financial support to patients with pancreatic cancer.

Fundraising for an Individual

There are many fundraising websites, each with its own special features. Some of these are GoFundMe, HelpHopeLive, CaringBridge, and GiveForward:

---

249. OpenAI. (2023). ChatGPT [Computer software]. Retrieved from https://www.openai.com/
250. Project Purple. (2023, August 10). Pancreatic cancer patient financial aid program. Retrieved from https://www.projectpurple.org/patients-families/patient-financial-aid/
251. National Pancreatic Cancer Foundation. (2023, August 7). Financial assistance. Retrieved from https://www.npcf.us/financial-assistance/

GoFundMe:

- Known worldwide, it's used for a variety of needs like medical bills, education fees, supporting charities, and personal goals.

- It offers tools to share your fundraising page on social media, which can help you reach many people fast.

- GoFundMe guides you on how to start and run your fundraising page and how to handle donations.

HelpHopeLive:

- This is a nonprofit group that helps people raise money for medical costs not covered by insurance, such as costs for a transplant, physical therapy, or special equipment.

- They check to make sure the money is really needed for medical reasons, and they give donors a receipt that can be used for tax deductions.

CaringBridge:

- This is a free service from a nonprofit group that lets people share news about their health with their friends and family.

- People can donate money directly to the person or family, and CaringBridge provides one-on-one help to guide you through the fundraising process.

GiveForward:

- This crowdfunding site focuses on helping people raise money for medical bills.

- They provide personal support and tools to help you raise money and do not charge a fee for personal fundraising pages.

It's a good idea to look at different medical fundraising websites and compare them to find the best one for your needs. Remember that each site has its rules, fees, and the type of people who use it, so choose the one that can help you and fits your specific situation.

When is a good time to start a fundraiser for someone in need?

Figuring out the best time to start a fundraiser for someone can be tough, and there's a lot to think about. You might wonder if it's a good idea to start a fundraiser. Here are some steps to help you decide when to start a fundraiser:

- First, see if the person is okay with starting a fundraiser and receiving money.

- Next, look at the person's money needs. Think about how much medical treatments and other expenses might cost.

- Think about other ways the person might find financial assistance. This could be from health insurance, government programs, or help from the local community.

- Also, think about how urgent the person's needs are. Like how soon they need surgery or a medical procedure.

- You should talk with experts like who know about fundraisers. They can help you make a good decision.

It's also important to make sure the fundraiser is fair and open. No one should get special treatment because they gave more money. Following these steps can help you decide how to start a fundraiser and how to run it.

Notoriety

Getting a famous person to help raise money for your medical care can be a great way to get more support. Here are some ideas on how to do it from AI:

1. **Friend of a Friend:** Maybe you know someone who knows a famous person. Ask your friend to introduce you or help pass along your message.

2. **Write a Letter:** Write a heartfelt letter explaining your situation and why you need help. Try to make it personal and real. You could send this letter through email or regular mail.

3. **Common Ground:** If you and a celebrity went to the same school or grew up in the same town, that's something you have in common! Sharing that in your letter could make them more interested in helping you.

4. **Shared Experience:** If a famous person or their family member has had the same disease or condition you have, they might feel a special connection to your cause. Reach out and share your story with them.

5. **Online Campaign:** You could start an online fundraising campaign and try to get it noticed by a celebrity. Use social media like Twitter, Instagram, or Facebook to spread your message.

6. **Local News:** You could also contact a local news outlet or radio station to share your story. If it gets enough attention, a celebrity might hear about it.

Remember, always be respectful and understanding. Not every famous person will be able or willing to help, and that's okay. Don't give up! Keep trying to approach different people, maybe in different ways, and you might find the support you need.[252]

Administering Funds and Who Should Help

When raising money for medical bills, it's important to pick someone you can trust to take care of the money. AI suggests a few different things that the person in charge should do to make sure the money is handled the right way:

- You should clearly plan how the money will be spent. It helps to have a special bank account just for the fundraiser money. This makes it easier to see where the money is going and helps to show everyone that everything is being done correctly.

- Keeping detailed records of all the money that comes in and goes out is also very important. Regular updates should be given to those who donated money so they know what's happening.

- If you collect a lot of money, consider getting help from a financial advisor. They can help make sure the money is managed correctly and follows all the legal rules related to taxes.

---

252. OpenAI. (2023). ChatGPT [Computer software]. Retrieved from https://www.openai.com/

- A financial advisor can advise on how to manage the money, including how to invest, what the tax rules are, and other money-related issues. They can also help make a plan for how to use the money.

- Lawyers can help with legal matters related to the fundraiser. For example, they can help understand rules related to charities, contracts, and any legal issues that might come up. They can also help write any legal documents that might be needed, like an agreement for the fundraiser.

- Accountants can help track the money and ensure all tax rules are followed. They are experts at preparing financial reports and filling out tax forms.

By getting advice from these professionals, you can make sure the money is managed properly and openly. But this is expensive and is only for very successful fundraisers. If you raise less than $25k, track and report it yourself. Between $25,000 and $100,000 hiring an accountant or, at least, a bookkeeper is a good idea. If you raise above $100,000, hiring an attorney (lawyer) and a financial advisor makes sense.[253]

This will help make sure the money is used in the best way for your medical needs. And when people see that everything is being done correctly, they may be more likely to donate.[254]

---

253. OpenAI. (2023). ChatGPT [Computer software]. Retrieved from https://www.openai.com/
254. OpenAI. (2023). ChatGPT [Computer software]. Retrieved from https://www.openai.com/

Free or Discounted Trips to Medical Centers

"My son's colleagues gave us airline and hotel points to use during our travel." **KH**

How to Start by AI:

1. **Talk to Your Doctor:** Ask your doctor to give you a letter explaining your condition and why you must travel. You should show this letter to the organization that can donate miles or points to you.

2. **Search for Organizations:** Find non-profit organizations that help people like you. Websites like Google can help. Search for phrases like "donated airline miles for medical patients" or "free hotel stays for cancer patients."

3. **Ask Your Social Worker:** If you have a social worker, they can greatly help find organizations. They often know where to look and whom to talk to.

4. **Fill Out Forms:** Once you find an organization or program, you'll usually need to fill out an application form. They might ask for a letter from your doctor and some other information.

5. **Wait for Approval:** After you send in your application, you might have to wait a little while. Each organization has its own rules, and it takes time for them to decide.

6. **Follow Up:** Don't be shy to follow up. Send an email or make a call to check your application's status.

7. **Say Thank You:** Remember to say thank you if you get the miles or points. These organizations love to hear how they've helped.

Where to Apply for Travel Help:

1. **Angel Flight:** "People Flying People in Need"

   Website: https://www.angelflight.com/

2. **Corporate Angel Network:** Helps cancer patients fly to treatment.

   Website: https://www.corpangelnetwork.org/

3. **Patient AirLift Services (PALS):** Provides free air travel for medical needs.

   Website: https://palservices.org/

4. **Southwest Airlines—Medical Transportation Grant Program:** Offers complimentary round-trip tickets to non-profit hospitals and medical transportation organizations.

   Website: https://www.southwest.com/citizenship/people/community-outreach/medical-transportation-grant-program/

5. **Miracle Flights:** Provides free commercial air travel to sick kids and adults who need out-of-state medical care.

   Website: https://miracleflights.org/

6. **Hawaiian Airlines:** Works with the American Cancer Society to transport people among the Hawaiian Islands for cancer treatment.

   Website: https://hphawaii.wordpress.com/2020/09/16/hawaiian-airlines-resumes-critical-transportation-for-cancer-patients/

7. **Airlines routinely allow individuals to transfer miles, and this is not limited to family members:** You may feel that asking someone (especially a business traveler) for airline miles is easier than asking them for money.

8. **Airlines that do not offer free travel directly to cancer patients:**

   A. Jet Blue (supports Angel Flight Northeast)

   B. Alaska Airlines (supports Angel Flight West)

   C. United Airlines (supports Fisher House)

   D. Delta Airlines

   E. American Airlines

9. **American Cancer Society Road to Recovery Program:**[255] "... provides transportation to and from treatment for people with cancer who do not have a ride or are unable to drive themselves."[256]

Website: https://www.cancer.org/support-programs-and-services/road-to-recovery.html

"Remember, programs have specific rules. For example, you might need to be a U.S. citizen, or you might need to be going to a specific type of treatment."[257]

Hotels/Lodging with Donation Programs:

1. **American Cancer Society Hope Lodge®:**

   - 500,000 nights of free lodging per year

   - 29,000 cancer patients and caregivers served per year

   - $55m lodging costs saved per year.

---

255. OpenAI. (2023). ChatGPT [Computer software]. Retrieved from https://www.openai.com/
256. American Cancer Society. (2023b). Road to recovery. Retrieved from https://www.cancer.org/support-programs-and-services/road-to-recovery.html
257. OpenAI. (2023). ChatGPT [Computer software]. Retrieved from https://www.openai.com/

- 6M nights of free lodging to cancer patients since 1970[258]

2. **Joe's House:** "We list cancer treatment centers and hospitals across the country with nearby lodging facilities that offer a discount."[259]

   Website: https://www.joeshouse.org/

3. **Healthcare Hospitality Network:** "Our House members provide lodging and support services to patients and their caregivers while they are receiving medical treatment away from their home communities."[260]

   Website: https://www.hhnetwork.org/about-us/

4. **Extended Stay America Partnership with the American Cancer Society:**

   For cancer patients, getting the right treatment sometimes requires traveling away from home. Lodging expenses can present a significant financial barrier to receiving lifesaving treatment, and financial barriers are known to contribute to disparities in cancer out-

---

258. American Cancer Society. (2023). American Cancer Society Hope Lodge: What is Hope Lodge? Retrieved from https://www.cancer.org/support-programs-and-services/patient-lodging/hope-lodge.html
259. Joe's House. (2023). Joe's House—A lodging guide for cancer patients. Retrieved from https://www.joeshouse.org/
260. Healthcare Hospitality Network. (2022, February 11). About us. Retrieved from https://www.hhnetwork.org/about-us/

comes. ... Extended Stay America has donated more than 150,000 hotel room nights.[261]

Website: https://www.extendedstayamerica.com/acs-partnership

5. **Fisher House Foundation:** "Fisher House Foundation builds comfort homes where military & veteran families can stay free of charge while a loved one is in the hospital."[262]

Website: https://fisherhouse.org/about/

Credit card companies and banks offer points for using their services, but these points usually don't directly help people who are sick with cancer. However, these companies and their customers donate money to various charities, and some of those charities help people with cancer.

What Non-Profits Offer

1. **Pancreatic Cancer Action Network (PanCAN)** advances research, clinical initiatives, patient services, and advocacy. They provide a range of services, including patient education, a clinical trial database, patient and caregiver support, and research grants. You can utilize PanCAN by

---

261. American Cancer Society. (2023a). American Cancer Society Patient Lodging Programs. Retrieved from https://www.cancer.org/support-programs-and-services/patient-lodging.html
262. Fisher House Foundation. (2023). About—Fisher House Foundation. Retrieved from https://fisherhouse.org/about/

participating in their advocacy efforts, attending or organizing fundraising events, or using their patient support resources.

Website: https://www.pancan.org/

2. **Let's Win** is an online forum for the entire pancreatic cancer community, including patients, families, doctors, and researchers. Among their recent highlights are:

- The launch of our reimagined website, now a trustworthy editorial platform with easy and more intuitive paths to information and resources.

- The return of an in-person benefit, where we honored Rich and Staci Grodin and remembered Juliette Gimon, the visionary behind the Survivor Video series.

- The publication of a paper confirming the power of our Twitter PancChat for reaching doctors and patients on social media.

- Further development of our partnerships, which allow us to broaden our reach into underserved communities.[263]

Website: https://letswinpc.org/

---

263. Let's Win Pancreatic Cancer. (2022, November 28). Annual report. https://letswinpc.org/about-us/annual-report/

3. **Lustgarten Foundation** is the largest private funder of pancreatic cancer research. They support research projects, facilitate collaborations among scientists, and work to advance early detection methods and more effective treatments. You can utilize the Lustgarten Foundation by contributing to fundraising, keeping informed about the latest research, or by applying for research grants if you're in the field.

   Website: https://lustgarten.org/

4. **Hirshberg Foundation for Pancreatic Cancer Research** funds pancreatic cancer research and provides patient education and support. They also host events to raise awareness and funds for pancreatic cancer. You can use the resources of the Hirshberg Foundation by attending their events, contributing to their fundraising efforts, or accessing their patient support resources.

   Website: https://www.pancreatic.org/

5. **National Pancreatic Cancer Foundation (NPCF)** provides direct financial assistance to pancreatic cancer patients and funds research into early detection methods. They also offer a nutritional program for patients undergoing treatment. You can utilize the NPCF by applying for financial aid if you're a patient or by contributing to their fundraising effort.

   Website: https://www.npcf.us/

6. **Rolfe Pancreatic Cancer Foundation** is dedicated to early detection research and patient support. They offer a free, personalized risk assessment tool on their website. You can utilize the Rolfe Foundation by accessing their risk assessment tool or by contributing to their fundraising and awareness campaigns.

   Website: https://www.rolfefoundation.org/

7. **The Sol Goldman Pancreatic Cancer Research Center** is a research center at Johns Hopkins University that focuses on pancreatic cancer research and clinical trials.

   "The Sol Goldman Pancreatic Cancer Research Center was established at Johns Hopkins in 2005 by the family of Sol and Lillian Goldman. This collaborative center supports cutting-edge pancreatic cancer research and hosts a thought-provoking annual Think Tank."[264]

   Website: https://pathology.jhu.edu/pancreas/sol-goldman-center

8. **Seena Magowitz Foundation** was founded in 2001 by Roger Magowitz to fund pancreatic cancer research after his mother was diagnosed with the disease. Today, the charity empowers the public with knowledge of pancreatic cancer and funds innovative research to find a cure.

---

264. The Sol Goldman Pancreatic Cancer Research Center. (2023). The Sol Goldman Pancreatic Cancer Research Center—Pancreatic Cancer | Johns Hopkins Pathology. Retrieved from https://pathology.jhu.edu/pancreas/sol-goldman-center

The Seena Magowitz Foundation funds clinical trials and pilot studies to develop innovative pancreatic cancer treatments. The charity then shares the latest research results with health care professionals and the public via their Pancreatic Cancer Podcast. In addition, the charity works to raise awareness of the disease by acting as a web-based information resource on the symptoms of pancreatic cancer, risk factors, and the types of treatment available.[265]

Website: http://www.seenamagowitzfoundation.org/

9. **National Pancreas Foundation** provides hope for those suffering from pancreatitis, pancreatic cancer, and FCS through funding cutting-edge research, advocating for new and better therapies, and providing support and education for patients, caregivers, and health care professionals.

To fulfill its mission, the National Pancreas Foundation provides research grants on an annual basis that are made directly to researchers to support ground-breaking research on pancreas disease. NPF is the only foundation dedicated to patients who are suffering from all forms of pancreas disease—pancreatic cancer, acute pancreatitis, chronic pancreatitis, pediatric pancreatitis, and FCS.

NPF and its Board of Directors and volunteers are committed to maximum efficiency, with over 93 cents of every dol-

---

[265]. Shaik, C. (2023, July 19). 9 best charities that fight pancreatic cancer (complete 2023 list). *Impactful Ninja*. Retrieved from https://impactful.ninja/best-charities-that-fight-pancreatic-cancer/

lar impacting patient programs and research, making NPF one of the most efficient charities in the United States.[266]

Website: https://pancreasfoundation.org/

10. **Family Reach** says 1 in 3 families facing cancer cannot meet their basic needs—food, housing, and transportation. Family Reach's services help patients cover everyday costs to access and adhere to cancer treatment.

23,247 families [were] supported in 2022. Our continuous measurement and evaluation help us understand where our funds go, how our support impacts cancer experiences, and whom we're reaching with our services.[267]

Website: https://familyreach.org/impact/

11. **American Cancer Society** was founded in 1913 by 10 doctors to raise public awareness of cancer. Today, the charity is a nationwide, community-based organization dedicated to eliminating all types of cancer, including pancreatic cancer. The American Cancer Society funds life-saving research into all forms of cancer, including pancreatic cancer. Through their American Cancer Society Action Network, the charity engages with elected officials to increase cancer prevention funding and improve access to health care for all Americans. In addition, the charity

---

266. National Pancreas Foundation. (2023, July 11). About—National Pancreas Foundation. Retrieved from https://pancreasfoundation.org/about/
267. Family Reach. (2023, September 7). Our impact: Helping cancer patients & caregivers. Retrieved from https://familyreach.org/impact/

offers cancer patient support through their 24-hour helpline. Through their community program services, the charity provides transport assistance, treatment referrals, and an online community platform for cancer patients.[268]

12. **Jessica Marulli Memorial Scholarship** Every year, this scholarship is given to college sophomores and juniors who focus on Liberal Arts & Social Sciences and have good grades, with at least a B average (3.0 GPA or higher). It's for students who really stand out because they have a unique hobby or passion in things like arts, music, or any specific area they love. This scholarship to Franklin Pierce University, the same university attended by Jessica's father, Al Marulli, making it a meaningful connection to their family's educational legacy.[269]

> Our mission is to change students' lives by awarding them an educational opportunity to better their future. In doing so, we honor and remember Jessica Marulli's legacy. A woman who shook the grounds she walked upon, and her courageous fight against pancreatic cancer. May Jessica's story impact these students, help shape them, guide them into a prosperous life.[270]

---

268. Shaik, C. (2023, July 19). 9 best charities that fight pancreatic cancer (complete 2023 list). *Impactful Ninja*. Retrieved from https://impactful.ninja/best-charities-that-fight-pancreatic-cancer/
269. The Jessica Marulli Memorial Scholarship. (n.d.). Retrieved January 10, 2024, from https://www.marullimemorialscholarship.com/
270. The Jessica Marulli Memorial Scholarship. (n.d.). Retrieved January 10, 2024, from https://www.marullimemorialscholarship.com/

Dip Into Your Rainy Day Fund

This book was written to be upbeat and give hope. But you know how people say that they are saving for a "rainy day"? Unfortunately, if you have pancreatic cancer, it's raining.

On the plus side that means it's time to do something special. You could go on a fun trip, give a present to someone special, or donate to a worthy cause you care about. Did you know that giving gifts often make you feel even happier than getting one?

Or maybe you've been dreaming about a cool car or something else you really want. You've waited a long time, so maybe now's the perfect moment to go for it. It's time to enjoy the things you've been saving up for.

Estate Planning

Estate planning is something everyone should think about. It means making plans for what will happen to your things after you're gone. It might be a bit scary to think about not being here, but don't worry. Thinking about it won't make the time come even a minute sooner.

So, what's the point of estate planning? Well, the main reason is that it legally allows you to choose what will happen to your money and debts after you pass away. With estate planning, you make the decisions. It's not left to chance or someone else. This way, your money goes to those people or causes you care most about. AI adds, "for example, you can choose to leave some money to your favorite charity or make sure your pet is taken care of."[271]

"This is a good time to get your affairs in order. You should review your estate plan and estate planning documents to ensure they are up to date and reflect your wishes." (Anonymous personal communication, January 30, 2024)

Medical Power of Attorney and Health Care Surrogate

If you have not already done so, you should execute a "medical power of attorney" and appointment of a "health care proxy". The purpose of these documents is to memorialize in writing the conditions under which you wish to remain alive and/or have life prolonging procedures or medications administered (among other things) and appoint the person(s) to carry out these wishes on your behalf. These documents come in a variety of names, forms and combinations, depending on the law of the state where you live. Other names for these documents may include Living Will, Health Care Proxy, Health Care Advance Directive, Advance Medical Directive, etc. You should provide your physician(s) with a copy of any such signed documents. (Anonymous personal communication, January 30, 2024)

---

271. OpenAI. (2023). ChatGPT [Computer software]. Retrieved from https://www.openai.com/

These legal papers are controlled by the laws of each state. If you're going to another state for medical treatment, bring them along. They might be useful. Even if they're not officially recognized, sharing your wishes can still be useful. If you're planning to have surgery in another state, it's smart to talk to the hospital or a lawyer about these papers a few weeks before your surgery.

Summary

"Do the best you can at the time you are doing it" are the words of my maternal grandmother, Evelina Carlson, which have helped inspire this book and my life. In a simple phrase, she motivates yet forgives an imperfect outcome, if you tried.

She would also encourage you to use "common sense." As defined by AI,

> Common sense is a simple but powerful concept that can be very helpful when we're dealing with tough or confusing situations. It's that inner voice or feeling that tells us what's right or wrong, safe or risky, based on what we already know. When we're scared or overwhelmed, as someone might be if they or a loved one is dealing with a serious illness like pancreatic cancer, emotions can cloud our thinking. That's why it's important to take a moment to pause and use common sense before making any big decisions.
>
> For example, if you're trying to decide on a treatment plan, using common sense might involve gathering all the information you can, talking to different doctors, and con-

sidering all the options before choosing the one that feels right for you. It might also involve talking to family and friends who can offer different perspectives and emotional support. In a way, using common sense is about balancing emotion with rational thought, so you can make the best choices possible.[272]

---

272. OpenAI. (2023). ChatGPT [Computer software]. Retrieved from https://www.openai.com/

Appendix A: Websites to Verify Medical Licenses

Alabama
https://www.albme.gov/consumers/licensee-search/

Alaska
https://www.commerce.alaska.gov/web/cbpl/Professional-Licensing/StateMedicalBoard/OnlineLicenseVerification.aspx

Arizona
https://azmd.gov/DoctorSearch/DoctorSearch/doctor-search
https://azbomprod.azmd.gov/glsuiteweb/clients/azbom/public/WebVerificationSearch.aspx

Arkansas
https://www.armedicalboard.org/public/verify/default.aspx

California
https://www.mbc.ca.gov/License-Verification/default.aspx

Colorado
https://www.medical-license-lookup.com/colorado/

Connecticut
https://www.elicense.ct.gov/Lookup/LicenseLookup.aspx

Delaware
https://delpros.delaware.gov/OH_VerifyLicense

Florida
https://mqa-internet.doh.state.fl.us/MQASearchServices/HealthCareProviders

Georgia
https://medicalboard.georgia.gov/verify-licensee

Hawaii
https://mypvl.dcca.hawaii.gov/public-license-search/

Idaho
https://apps-dopl.idaho.gov/IBOMPublic/LPRBrowser.aspx

Illinois
https://online-dfpr.micropact.com/lookup/licenselookup.aspx

Indiana
https://indiana.licenselookup.org/medical/

Iowa
https://medicalboard.iowa.gov/applyrenew-license/verifications

Kansas
https://www.kansas.gov/ksbn-verifications/search/records

Kentucky
http://web1.ky.gov/GenSearch/LicenseSearch.aspx?AGY=5

Louisiana
https://online.lasbme.org/#/verifylicense

Maine
https://www.maine.gov/md/licensure/license-verification

Maryland
https://www.mbp.state.md.us/mbp_ah/verification.aspx

Massachusetts
https://www.mass.gov/info-details/check-a-health-profession-license
https://massachusetts.licenselookup.org/medical/

Michigan
https://michigan.licenselookup.org/medical/
https://www.michigan.gov/lara/i-need-to/find-or-verify-a-licensed-professional-or-business

Minnesota
https://bmp.hlb.state.mn.us/#/onlineEntitySearch

Mississippi
https://gateway.licensure.msbn.ms.gov/Verification/search.aspx

Missouri
https://pr.mo.gov/licensee-search-division.asp

Montana
https://ebizws.mt.gov/PUBLICPORTAL/searchform?mylist=licenses
https://boards.bsd.dli.mt.gov/medical-examiners/

Nebraska
https://www.nebraska.gov/LISSearch/search.cgi

Nevada
https://nsbme.us.thentiacloud.net/webs/nsbme/register/

New Hampshire
https://forms.nh.gov/licenseverification/

New Jersey
https://newjersey.mylicense.com/verification/Search.aspx

New Mexico
http://docfinder.docboard.org/nm/

New York
https://www.health.ny.gov/professionals/doctors/conduct/license_lookup.htm

North Carolina
https://portal.ncmedboard.org/verification/search.aspx

North Dakota
https://www.ndbom.org/public/find_verify/verify.asp

Ohio
https://elicense.ohio.gov/OH_HomePage

Oklahoma
https://www.okmedicalboard.org/search

Oregon
https://omb.oregon.gov/search

Pennsylvania
https://www.pals.pa.gov/#!/page/search

Rhode Island
https://healthri.mylicense.com/verification/

South Carolina
https://verify.llronline.com/LicLookup/Med/Med.aspx

South Dakota
https://login.sdbmoe.gov/Public/Services/VerificationSearch

Tennessee
https://apps.health.tn.gov/licensure/default.aspx

Texas
https://public.tmb.state.tx.us/HCP_Search/SearchNotice.aspx

Utah
https://secure.utah.gov/llv/search/index.html

Vermont
https://mpb.health.vermont.gov/Lookup/LicenseLookup.aspx

Virginia
https://dhp.virginiainteractive.org/Lookup/Index

Washington
https://fortress.wa.gov/doh/providercredentialsearch/

West Virginia
https://wvbom.wv.gov/public/search/

Wisconsin
https://licensesearch.wi.gov/

Wyoming
https://wyomedboard.wyo.gov/consumers/license-lookup
https://wybomprod.glsuite.us/GLSuiteWeb/Clients/WYBOM/Public/Licenseesearch.aspx

Appendix B: Definitions and Abbreviations

Amino acids: Just like cement blocks are used to build walls, amino acids are what make up proteins. Think of DNA like a set of blueprints (building instructions) that tell where each of the 20 different kinds of amino acids should go. When amino acids are put together in a specific order, they make a protein that has a special job in the body.

It's kind of like when you use cement blocks to build a house. The way you arrange the blocks will decide what the house will be like and how it will be used. The order of amino acids decides what a protein will do.

CT (computerized tomography): A CT scan is like a super-advanced x-ray. Regular x-rays give you just one flat picture, but a CT scan takes lots of x-rays from different angles. Then, a computer puts all these pictures together to make a 3D image. This way, doctors can see inside your body from all sides and get a much better idea of what's going on.

DNA (deoxyribonucleic acid): It's the instruction manual for all the cells in your body. DNA is made of special molecules that form genes, which tell the cells what to do. When something goes wrong with the DNA, as in pancreatic cancer, it can cause big problems. DNA is really, really complicated. If scientists, perhaps through AI, learn more about it and find ways to fix or change it, we could get better at finding and treating pancreatic cancer early.

Enzymes: These are special kinds of protein, and you can think of them like robots in a factory. Each enzyme has one specific job, and it keeps doing that job over and over again. Another kind of enzyme, called a cell receptor, works like a doorbell for cells. When a hormone, which is like a messenger in the body, shows up, the cell receptor lets the cell know.

There are hundreds of thousands of different jobs that enzymes do in our bodies. If we can understand the enzymes that aren't working right in pancreatic cancer, we might find better ways to treat it. So, studying these enzymes gives us hope for better treatments in the future.

Endoscopic ultrasound: This is a special way doctors can get pictures of your pancreas. They use sound waves to make these images. Because your pancreas is deep inside your body, they have to get the sound wave equipment really close to it. They will give you a mild dose of sleeping medicine so you won't feel uncomfortable during the procedure. Then the doctor will insert a tube through your mouth and into your stomach. This is safe and common procedure.

This tube has a probe that sends out sound waves and a microphone that catches the echoes of those sound waves. This helps take a picture of your pancreas.

IV (intravenous line): This is a small rubber tube that goes directly into your vein to give you medicine or special saltwater to keep you hydrated. There are two main kinds of IVs:

Peripheral: This one goes into a small vein, usually in your arm. It's used for a short time, like a few hours to a couple of days. Doctors use it to give you things like antibiotics or fluids to keep you hydrated. To put it in, they use a needle, but then they take the needle out and only the tube stays in your vein. Sometimes, it can feel a little weird when you move, like the needle is still there, but it's not.

Central: The one used for chemo is called a Port-A-Cath. It is put into a large vein, usually one near your collarbone, during a small surgery. It has a round part, like the top of a drum, that stays under your skin. This type of IV can stay in for months without causing much, if any, discomfort. Doctors use it to give really strong medicines like chemotherapy, which has to go into a big vein because it would harm a small vein.

Each type of IV has its own uses and reasons, and both are important tools for doctors to help treat people.

Insurance Preauthorization: Insurance preauthorization is like asking for permission from your insurance company before you get a medical treatment, test, or buy medicine. It's a way to make sure the insurance company will help pay for them. It is also a way that health insurers control their costs.[273]

Metastatic Cancer: Cancer that has spread by way of the bloodstream or lymphatic channels to distant parts of the body. Note that metastatic cancer still has the properties of the original cancer regardless of location. For instance, pancreatic cancer that has metastasized to the liver is still pancreatic cancer, not liver cancer.

MRCP (magnetic resonance cholangiopancreatography): An MRI with IV dye used to make detailed images of the pancreas, pancreatic duct, liver, gallbladder, and bile duct.

MRI or MR (magnetic resonance imaging): An imaging technique that uses a strong magnetic field but no radiation to produce computer-generated, three-dimensional pictures of the body.

Palliative Care: Palliative care (pronounced PAL-lee-uh-tiv) is specialized medical care for people with serious illness. This type of care is focused on providing relief from the symptoms such as pain, nausea, constipation and fatigue. Care providers aim to reduce the stress of serious illness. The goal is to improve the quality of life for both the patient and the family.

Palliative care is provided by a specially trained team of doctors, nurses, and other specialists who work together with a

---

273. OpenAI. (2023). ChatGPT [Computer software]. Retrieved from https://www.openai.com/

patient's other doctors to provide an extra layer of support. It is appropriate at any age and at any stage in a serious illness, and it can be provided along with curative treatment.[274]

RNA (ribonucleic acid): A chemical the body uses in the process of taking the information stored in DNA to make proteins. Not all genes in each cell are being used at any one time. The presence of RNA specific to a gene means that gene is active. Think of the "R" in RNA as a "receipt" for the use of a gene. Testing for RNA is much more expensive than testing for DNA, but it offers hope for the diagnosis and treatment of pancreatic cancer.

PERT (pancreatic enzyme replacement therapy): Oral supplements to help you digest food when your pancreas is not functioning properly or has been removed by surgery.

Protein: Think of proteins as the buildings of the body. Just as there are many different types of buildings (homes, factories, stores, etc.), there are proteins that serve a vast variety of functions in the body (structure, muscle, enzymes, and cell markers). Again, proteins are made from unique combinations of about twenty amino acids, the way buildings are made from cement blocks.

Targeted therapy: Targeted therapy is a type of cancer treatment that's personalized for you. It works by first studying what's unique about your cancer. Then, based on these find-

---

274. Get Palliative Care. (n.d.). What is Palliative Care? Retrieved July 25, 2023, from https://getpalliativecare.org/whatis/

ings, doctors create specific treatments that target those unique aspects. This way, the treatment can be more effective in fighting your cancer.

Afterword

Dr. Campazzi's requests

If possible, donate some of your cancer cells for an organoid. Donating cells for organoids can be done in a few ways. You can give a small piece of tissue through a biopsy of your pancreas. If your cancer has spread to your liver, it can be biopsied. You can also offer a part of tissue removed during surgery, or choose an easier method like a liquid biopsy, where you just need to give a blood sample. An organoid may well improve your care and outcome. If not, it will help others.

If my book helped you, please post a review on Amazon. If you read a free copy, please buy one, as only reviews from verified purchasers count. You could **pay it forward** by giving the extra copy to your oncologist for the next patient. This will help me write my next book.

About the Intern

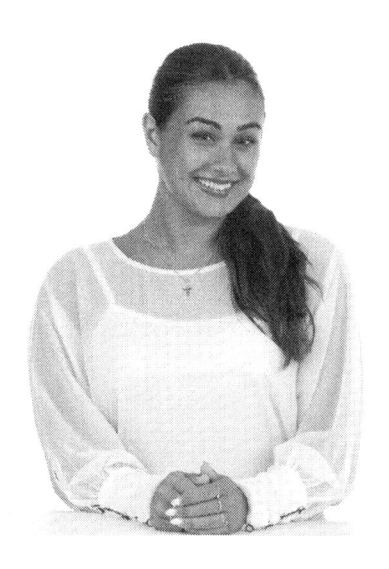

Guilianna "Jules" Johnston is a student athlete and sophomore at Rice University. She has an A average while playing Division 1 collegiate soccer for the 2022 Conference USA champions, the Rice Owls.

Jules attended Suncoast High School, which ranks in the country's top 50 best magnet schools. She set the Palm Beach County record for scoring 63 goals in a single season.

Jules is planning a career in medicine, majoring in Kinesiology, because she has always had an immense desire to work in the medical field. Her fascination with anatomy and the intricate workings of the human body intensified as she moved through school, sparking her interest in learning more about the underlying processes behind wellness and sickness. To Jules, entering the medical field is not just a career choice; it is a lifelong commitment to assist, heal, and uplift others. She is ecstatic to embark on this challenging and rewarding journey in her near future.

About the Author

Dr. Earl J. Campazzi, Jr. is a primary care physician with a concierge medicine practice in Palm Beach, Florida. He is highly educated, with 11 years of study beyond college, and many patients have thanked him for his medical care. Dr. Campazzi is deeply gratified and humbled by several patients having told him that his care has saved their lives. He has certifications in four areas of medicine: preventive medicine, occupational medicine, hospice/palliative medicine, and medical informatics, which involves managing and communicating medical information.

He has studied and worked at several of the best medical centers in the country. He used to work at the Mayo Clinic in Rochester, Minnesota. There, he helped take care of their employees, including other doctors. He also taught at the Mayo Clinic School of Medicine. He finished his medical training at Johns Hopkins and was picked to be the top physician in his class, Chief Resident.

Dr. Campazzi went to the University of Pittsburgh School of Medicine to become a doctor. After that, he earned more degrees. From Johns Hopkins University, he has a Master of Public Health degree, where he focused on healthcare policy and management. He also has a Master of Health Sciences degree in immunology and infectious diseases from Johns Hopkins. He received his Master of Business Administration degree from Duke University Fuqua School of Business, focusing on health services management. His Bachelor of Arts degree also came from the Johns Hopkins University.

Dr. Campazzi lives in West Palm Beach, Florida, with his wife, Julie. They enjoy a little travel, occasional golf, and especially dinners with friends. Julie wrote a fun time-travel book about mythical Greece for middle school kids. They have three dogs named Buster, Fred, and Lilly, who are a breed called Chinese Crested Powderpuffs.

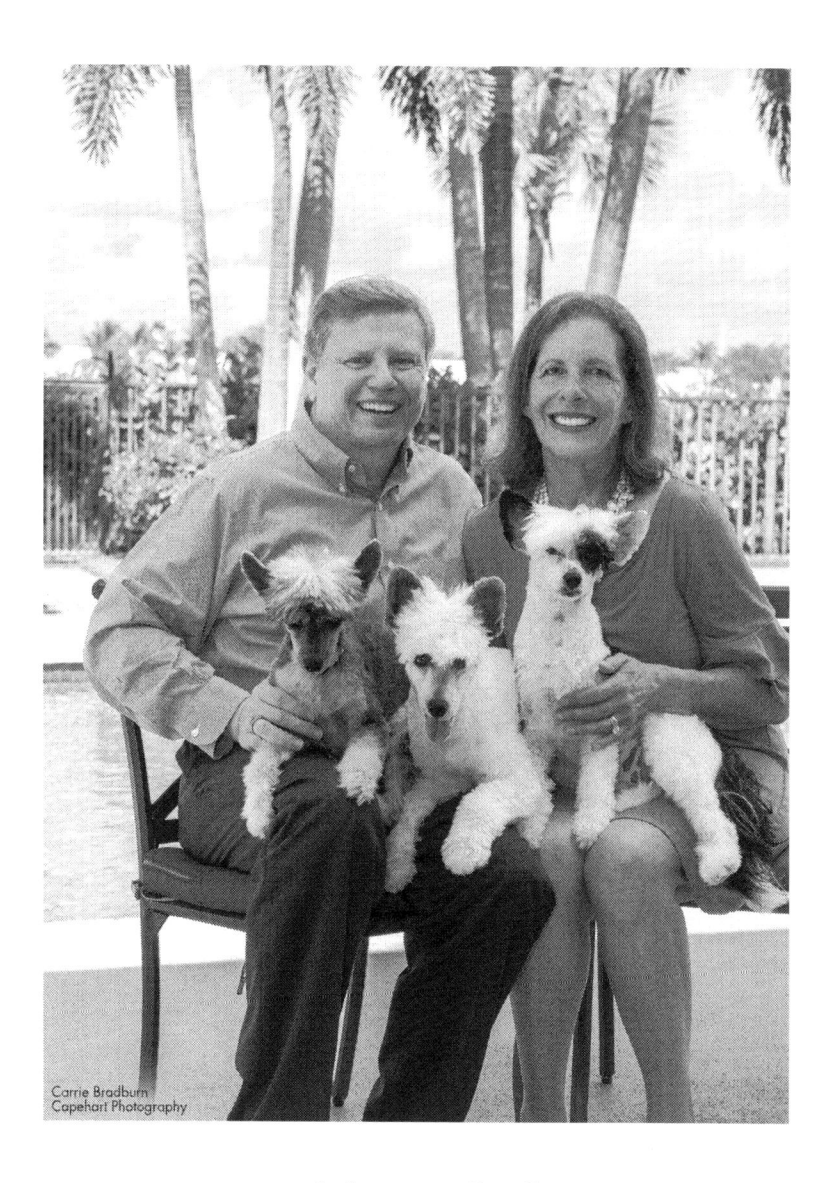

Living with Pancreatic Cancer: A Patient and Family Guide

Carrie Bradburn
Capehart Photography

We wish you the best!

Made in the USA
Columbia, SC
21 May 2024